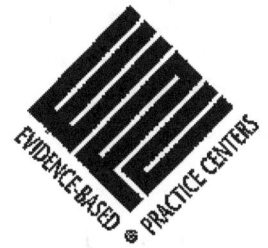

Measuring Health-Related Quality of Life for Patients with Diabetic Retinopathy

Technology Assessment Report

Project ID: DBTR0610

April 23, 2012

University of Alberta Evidence-based Practice Center

Andrea Milne, B.ScN., M.L.I.S.
Jeffery A. Johnson B.S.P., M.Sc., Ph.D.
Matthew Tennant, B.A., M.D., F.R.C.S.C., Dip. A.B.O.
Christopher Rudnisky, M.D., M.P.H., F.R.C.S.C.
Donna M. Dryden, Ph.D.

This report is based on research conducted by the University of Alberta Evidence-based Practice Center under contract to the Agency for Healthcare Research and Quality (AHRQ), Rockville, MD (Contract No. HHSA 290 2007 10021 I). The findings and conclusions in this document are those of the author(s) who are responsible for its contents; the findings and conclusions do not necessarily represent the views of AHRQ. No statement in this article should be construed as an official position of the Agency for Healthcare Research and Quality or of the U.S. Department of Health and Human Services.

The information in this report is intended to help health care decision-makers; patients and clinicians, health system leaders, and policymakers, make well-informed decisions and thereby improve the quality of health care services. This report is not intended to be a substitute for the application of clinical judgment. Decisions concerning the provision of clinical care should consider this report in the same way as any medical reference and in conjunction with all other pertinent information, i.e., in the context of available resources and circumstances presented by individual patients.

This report may be used, in whole or in part, as the basis for development of clinical practice guidelines and other quality enhancement tools, or as a basis for reimbursement and coverage policies. AHRQ or U.S. Department of Health and Human Services endorsement of such derivative products may not be stated or implied.

Andrea Milne, Jeffery A, Johnson and Donna M. Dryden have no affiliations or financial involvement related to the material presented in this report. Drs. Matthew Tennant and Christopher Rudnisky are directors of and have financial interests in Secure Diagnostic Imaging Inc., a company that developed and manages teleophthalmology software for the diagnosis and followup of diabetic retinopathy. There is no treatment performed via the software. Therefore, there is no conflict with their role in the development of, or the material presented in this report. Drs. Tennant and Rudnisky provided clinical expertise to the University of Alberta research team, feedback on draft reports, and assisted in writing background material on diabetic retinopathy.

Acknowledgments

The authors gratefully acknowledge the following individuals for their contributions to this project: Kenneth Bond for the protocol development and level one screening, Kelly Russell for level one and level two screening, Elizabeth Sumamo for level one and level two screening, Christine Ha for data abstraction and verification, Carol Spooner for quality assessment, Annabritt Chisholm for article retrieval, and Jennifer Seida for copyediting.

Peer Reviewers

We wish to acknowledge individuals listed below for their review of this report. This report has been reviewed in draft form by individuals chosen for their expertise and diverse perspectives. The purpose of the review was to provide candid, objective, and critical comments for consideration by the EPC in preparation of the final report. Synthesis of the scientific literature presented here does not necessarily represent the views of individual reviewers.

Jerry Cavallerano
Department of Ophthalmology, Harvard Medical School,
Beetham Eye Institute, Joslin Diabetes Center
Boston, Massachusetts

Theodore Leng
Clinical Assistant Professor
Byers Eye Institute at Stanford
Palo Alto, California

Deborah Wexler
Assistant Professor
MGH and Harvard Medical School
Boston, Massachusetts

Ingrid Zimmer-Galler
Associate Professor
Johns Hopkins Wilmer Eye Institute
Baltimore, Maryland

Structured Abstract

Objectives: To identify and evaluate the psychometric properties of tools used to measure health-related quality of life (HRQL) in patients receiving treatment for diabetic retinopathy (DR), and to assess the effectiveness of interventions for DR to improve HRQL.

Data Sources: We conducted a systematic and comprehensive search in six electronic databases and hand searched reference lists of reviews and included studies.

Review Methods: Study selection, quality assessment, and data extraction were completed by reviewers independently and in duplicate. We included articles that presented data on HRQL outcomes following an intervention for DR (including diabetic macular edmema (DME). Mean differences and 95 percent confidence intervals were calculated for continuous outcomes. We did not conduct any meta-analyses due to heterogeneity.

Results: We identified four validated HRQL measures: 36–Item Short Form Health Survey (SF–36), National Eye Institute Visual Functioning Questionnaire (VFQ–25 and –51), Visual Function Index (VF–14), and Diabetes Treatment Satisfaction Questionnaire (DTSQ). We also identified two tools that are currently undergoing evaluation: the Retinopathy Treatment Satisfaction Questionnaire (RetTSQ) and the Retinopathy Dependent Quality of Life (RetDQoL).

Two randomized controlled trials (RCTs) reported on HRQL outcomes following anti-vascular endothelial growth factor (anti-VEGF) treatment for DME. Seven observational studies reported on HRQL outcomes following: laser photocoagulation (two), vitrectomy (two), panretinal photocoagulation versus vitrectomy (one), and phacoemulsification cataract surgery (two).

The RCT comparing pegaptanib sodium versus sham reported a statistically significant improvement from baseline for the composite score of the VFQ–25 at 2 years (but not at 1 year). The three-arm RCT comparing ranibizumab monotherapy versus ranibizumab plus laser versus laser showed a statisitically significant difference for the composite score of the VFQ–25 for both anti-VEGF arms versus laser at 1 year. The strength of evidence for anti-VEGF was assessed as low.

For the remaining interventions, the studies were at high risk of bias due to weak study designs (before-after and cohort studies) and poor implementation. There is insufficient evidence to determine whether one of these treatments for DR is more effective than another in improving HRQL in this patient population.

Conclusions: We identified few HRQL measurement instruments that have been used to assess the impact of treatment in patients with DR or DME; however, the tools that have been used have been adequately evaluated. Two tools developed specifically for patients with DR are currently undergoing evaluation. In general, HRQL was improved following interventions for DR. Further research on HRQL following anti-VEGF treatment for DME is needed to confirm the results of two RCTs. The current research on the impact of other interventions for DR on HRQL is insufficient to draw conclusions about the relative effect of one intervention versus another. RCTs that assess the impact of treatments for DR should include HRQL as an outcome.

Contents

Executive Summary 1
Introduction 1
   Diabetic Retinopathy 1
   Health-Related Quality of Life 2
      Patient-Reported Outcomes 2
      Health Status/Functional Status 2
      Health-Related Quality of Life/Quality of Life 2
      Measuring Health-Related Quality of Life/Quality of Life 3
      Psychometric Properties for HRQL Tools 4
   Key Questions 5
   Analytic Framework 6
Methods 8
   Literature Search 8
   Study Selection 8
      Study Design 8
      Population 8
      Intervention and comparator 9
      Outcome 9
   Data Extraction 9
   Assessment of Methodological Quality 9
      Quality Assessment of HRQL Tools 9
      Quality Assessment for Included Studies 9
   Data Analysis 10
   Grading the Evidence for Question 2 10
Results 11
   Literature Review and Screening 11
   Generic Assessment Tools 13
      Medical Outcomes Study (MOS) 36–Item Short Form Health Survey (SF–36) 13
   Low-Vision Related Assessment Tools 14
      National Eye Institute Visual Function Questionnaire-25-item version (VFQ–25) .. 14
      Visual Function–14 (VF–14) 14
   Diabetes-Related HRQL Assessment Tools 14
      Diabetes Treatment Satisfaction Questionnaire (DTSQ) 14
   Diabetic Retinopathy Related HRQL Assessment Tools 15
      Diabetic Retinopathy Dependent Quality of Life (RetDQoL) 15
      Diabetic Retinopathy Treatment Satisfaction Questionnaire (RetTSQ) 15
   Description of Included Studies 22
   Methodological Quality 22
   Results 23
      Laser photocoagulation 23
      Vitrectomy 24
      Vitrectomy and panretinal photocoagulation 25
      Phacoemulsifcation 25
   Summary of Findings 30

    HRQL Measures 32
    Impact of interventions on HRQL 33
  Recommendations for Future Research 33
  Conclusions 34
References 34
Abbreviations and Acronyms 35

Tables

Table 1. Psychometric properties of health-related quality of life assessment tools used in studies of the treatment of diabetic retinopathy 16
Table 2. Rating of the psychometric properties health-related quality of life assessment tools used in studies of treatment of diabetic retinopathy 21
Table 3. Study characteristics and outcomes for studies reporting the impact of interventions for diabetic retinopathy on HRQL 27
Table 4. Strength of evidence for health-related quality of life outcomes 31

Figures

Figure 1. Analytic Framework. 7
Figure 2. Flow-diagram for Study Retrieval and Selection. 12

Appendixes

Appendix A. Search Strategies
Appendix B. Inclusion/Exclusion Form
Appendix C. List of excluded studies
Appendix D. Characteristics of the health-related quality of life assessment tools used in studies of the treatment of diabetic retinopathy
Appendix E. Sample health-related quality of life assessment tools
Appendix F. Extended study characteristics and outcomes for studies reporting the impact of interventions for diabetic retinopathy on health-related quality of life

Executive Summary

Introduction

Diabetic Retinopathy

Diabetic retinopathy (DR) is a leading cause of vision loss in the United States and occurs as a result of pathologic changes of the retinal vasculature.[1] In 2005–2008, the estimated crude prevalence among Americans over the age of 40 with diabetes was 28.5 percent. Although the prevalence of vision-threatening DR is approximately 4.4 percent,[2] the number of affected Americans 40 years or older is expected to triple from 1.2 million in 2005 to 3.4 million in 2050.[3] The prevalence and severity of DR increases with the duration of diabetes; however, it is inversely correlated to glycemic and blood pressure control.[4,5] Moderate vision loss is most commonly related to retinal leakage within the macula, while severe vision loss usually occurs as a result of neovascularization (proliferative diabetic retinopathy; PDR) with subsequent hemorrhage or fibrosis.[6]

Early identification and treatment of DR is important since treatment is both cost-effective and reduces vision loss.[7] The American Academy of Ophthalmologists, the American Optometric Association, and the American Diabetes Association recommend an annual dilated eye examination for all people with diabetes, and more frequent eye examinations for people with known DR.[8-10] Other researchers argue that the frequency of examinations should be stratified to an individual's risk of progression and vision loss.[11]

The mainstay of DR treatment is aimed at reducing the risk of onset and limiting the progression of the disease. Therefore, retinal assessments should be performed on a regular basis to determine the presence and degree of DR, glycemic control should be optimized, and known risk factors such as blood pressure, dyslipidemia, elevated cholesterol, renal disease and abdominal obesity should be controlled. Direct ocular therapy should be prescribed when indicated, while vision rehabilitation and low vision aids should to be used to maximize vision if there is a loss.[4,5]

Until recently, the primary treatment for DR has been focal or grid laser of the retina.[12,13] Serial intravitreal injections of triamcinolone have been introduced as a treatment option as they have been shown to be effective at reducing diabetic macular edema (DME); however, their use is becoming less common due to significant adverse effects including elevated intraocular pressure and cataract formation.[14,15] Ranibizumab and becvacizumab are being used with increasing frequency for the treatment of DME; however they have not yet been approved for use in this condition by the Food and Drug Administration. The recommended treatment of PDR remains panretinal photocoagulation[16] with vitrectomy surgery performed when necessary.[14] It is important to note that treatment of DR is not always aimed at restoration of pre-disease visual acuity, but rather at limiting further deterioration. Patients may report a decrease in visual acuity immediately after therapy, which may manifest in low initial perceptions of treatment satisfaction. However, results from the Early Treatment Diabetic Retinopathy Study demonstrate that early treatment with either panretinal photocoagulation or vitrectomy prevents long-term disability due to blindness.[12-14]

Diabetic patients with retinopathy have reported that vision loss impacts multiple areas of well-being including: independence, mobility, leisure, and self-care.[7,17,18] Additionally, DR has been found to impair functioning and overall health-related quality of life (HRQL).[19,20]

Health Related Quality of Life

Patient Reported Outcomes. Patient reported outcomes (PROs) measure a variety of aspects of care including HRQL, patient illness perceptions, and treatment satisfaction or adherence.[21] PROs are distinguished from other outcomes because the report is from the patient's perspective, usually without interpretation by another individual.[22] PROs include: health status, functional status, and quality of life (QOL) or HRQL.[23,24] Health status refers to the identification and assessment of the changes in patients' activities and perceptions compared with normal life.[24] Functional status focuses on the physical capacity to complete everyday activities at home or work. QOL covers a range of experiences related to patients' well-being based on their subjective experiences.[25] Many variables, both objective and subjective, interact to define QOL,[26] but it is dependent upon individual patient experiences, states, and perceptions of their illness.[25] HRQL allows clinicians and researchers to measure the impact of chronic diseases such as diabetes mellitus on the lives of patients.[23] It takes into account the impact of disease and its treatments on physical, psychological, social, and somatic domains of functioning and well-being.[25]

Measuring Health-Related Quality of Life/Quality of Life. Collecting HRQL and QOL outcomes allows clinicians and researchers to take into account a wider array of information that cannot be obtained through laboratory or physical measures, and provides a subjective description of functioning alongside objective findings.[27] Through the collection of patient perceptions of interventions, health care providers can better understand what aspects of health patients value most highly and therefore what types of treatment may provide the greatest benefit.

Just as the definitions of HRQL and QOL vary, so too do the tools used for evaluating these outcomes. Evaluation tools may be as simple as a single question asking patients to state their QOL; however, they are more likely to take the form of a questionnaire with multiple items that investigate different domains related to HRQL.[23] HRQL tools can be divided into two categories: generic instruments and specific instruments.

Generic HRQL tools investigate all important aspects of HRQL and allow broad comparisons, but do not necessarily investigate a specific aspect of disease.[28] These tools may be less responsive to change as they provide an overall summary score of HRQL.[23] Specific HRQL instruments target a particular disease, population, or an outcome. Where generic tools allow broad comparisons, specific tools may be more responsive to HRQL changes in the specific patient population under investigation.[23]

Psychometric Properties for HRQL Tools. The large number of HRQL tools that are available can make it difficult for researchers and clinicians to determine what tools are the most trustworthy and appropriate for use in clinical and research settings. In recent years, a group of international researchers has undertaken the challenge of identifying what psychometric properties are of greatest importance when evaluating the quality of a HRQL tool, and what criteria should be used in judging the psychometric properties. In 2010, the COnsensus-based Standards for the selection of health Measurement INstruments (COSMIN) checklist was released for the purpose of evaluating the methodological quality of studies investigating the psychometric properties of HRQL tools.[29] The COSMIN researchers also reached consensus on definitions for these psychometric properties (Table ES1).

Table ES1. Definitions of psychometric properties

Domain	Psychometric Property	Definition
Reliability		Reliability is the degree to which the tool is free from measurement error.
	Internal Consistency	Internal consistency reliability is a reflection of the reproducibility of measurement by different items within a multi-item scale.
	Test-retest Reliability	Test-retest reliability is the degree to which the score of a patient who has not changed remains the same under repeated measurements.
Validity		Validity is defined as the degree to which an instrument measures the construct(s) it is intended to measure.
	Content Validity	Content validity is concerned with the content of the measurement tool and whether it is an adequate reflection of the construct to be measured.
	Construct Validity	Construct validity considers whether the scores produced by the instrument are consistent with the hypothesis of how the tool should behave, assuming the tool is valid.
	Criterion Validity	Criterion validity focuses on the degree to which the scores of an instrument reflect a 'gold standard'.
Responsiveness		The responsiveness of a tool demonstrates the ability of the instrument to detect changes in a patient over time when changes in the construct being measured actually occur.
Interpretability		Interpretability is considered important for the usability of the measurement tool rather than as a psychometric property. It is the degree to which a clinician or researcher can equate a qualitative meaning to an instrument's quantitative score.

Key Questions

1a. What HRQL measures have been used in studies of treatments for DR?

1b. What are the psychometric properties of the HRQL measures used in the studies?

2. Including only studies that have used reliable and valid measures, what is the evidence that HRQL is improved for any intervention for DR? What is the comparative effectiveness of interventions to improve HRQL in patients with DR?

3. What evidence is presented in the studies about the relationship between the measured improvement in HRQL and any relevant variables, including but not limited to baseline visual acuity, age (≥65 years), race, sex, severity, and type of DR (i.e., DME, nonproliferative diabetic retinopathy (NPDR), PDR)?

Methods

Literature Search

We conducted systematic and comprehensive searches in the following databases: MEDLINE®, EMBASE®, PsychINFO®, Cochrane Central Register of Controlled Trials®, CINAHL Plus full text, and Scopus to identify relevant studies to address the Key Questions. The searches were run in July 2010. An update search including PubMed was run in March 2011. A full search update was run in January 2012. No date or language restrictions were applied. We also conducted a search of ClinicalTrials.gov for recently completed or ongoing studies. To supplement the database searches, we hand searched the reference lists of review articles and included studies. We did not search for conference papers.

Study Selection

Two reviewers independently screened titles and abstracts using broad inclusion criteria. The full text of articles identified as "include" or "unclear" were retrieved for formal review. Each article was independently assessed by two reviewers using detailed a priori inclusion criteria and a standardized form. Disagreements were resolved by consensus or by third party adjudication, as needed.

For all questions the population of interest was adults (≥18 years) with DR including DME, NPDR, PDR, and other related conditions. For Key Question 1, we included studies that reported the use of any measurement tool that included at least one domain of HRQL, and we considered all study designs. For Key Questions 2 and 3, we included prospective comparative studies that investigated any intervention. We included studies that used a HRQL measurement tool with published data on the instrument's psychometric properties. There were no language restrictions. We excluded studies that were only available as abstracts.

Quality Assessment and Grading the Body of Evidence

Quality Assessment of HRQL Tools. We used the COSMIN[29,36] checklist to evaluate the psychometric properties of HRQL instruments. The following domains were assessed: content and construct validity, internal consistency, reliability, absolute measurement error, responsiveness, and interpretability.[37] Each domain was rated as "no data available," "low quality," "indeterminate," or "high quality." One reviewer assessed the HRQL tools in consultation with an expert in the HRQL field.

Quality Assessment of Included Studies. We assessed trials using the Cochrane Risk of Bias (ROB) tool for randomized controlled trials (RCTs).[38] The ROB includes six domains which assess sequence generation, allocation concealment, blinding (participants and personnel, and outcome assessors), incomplete outcome data, selective outcome reporting, and other sources of bias.

We assessed cohort studies using a modified version of the Newcastle-Ottawa Scale (NOS) for cohort studies.[39] The NOS includes seven items assessing sample selection, comparability of cohorts, and the assessment of outcomes. The methodological quality of before-after studies was assessed using the modified NOS that assessed sample selection and the assessment of outcomes. Two reviewers independently assessed the methodological quality; discrepancies were resolved through consensus or third party adjudication, as needed.

Grading the Evidence for Question 2. The overall strength of evidence for HRQL was assessed using the EPC GRADE approach.[40] The following four domains were examined: risk of bias (including study design and study conduct), consistency, directness, and precision. The overall strength of evidence was graded as "high," "moderate," "low," or "insufficient." One reviewer rated the strength of evidence.

Data Abstraction and Analysis

One reviewer extracted data directly into evidence tables, and a second reviewer checked the data for accuracy and completeness. Disagreements were resolved through discussion or third party adjudication, as needed.

We calculated mean differences and 95 percent confidence intervals (95% CI) for continuous variables. We did not conduct any meta-analysis due to the heterogeneity of interventions and patient characteristics.

Results

Literature Review

The electronic literature search identified 6,961 unique citations. Sixteen studies addressed Key Question 1a. Of these, 11 used validated HRQL measures (Key Question 1b). Nine primary studies provided data to address Key Questions 2 and 3.

Key Question 1a. What HRQL measures have been used in studies of treatments for diabetic retinopathy?

We identified four HRQL measures that have been used in studies assessing the treatment of DR. The most commonly used measure was the National Eye Institute Visual Functioning Questionnaire (VFQ). Five studies[41,42,45-47] used the 25-item version (VFQ–25); one[48] used the 51 item version (VFQ–51). In addition, seven recently completed trials that have not yet published their results reported using the VFQ–25. One study[49] used both the VFQ–25 and the Medical Outcomes Study (MOS) 36–Item Short Form Health Survey (SF–36). Two studies[46,47] used the Visual Function Index (VF–14). One study used both the VF–14 and the MOS 12–Item Short Form Health Survey (SF–12),[52] and another study[53] used the VF–14 plus a questionnaire to assess satisfaction with surgical outcomes. One study[54] used the Diabetes Treatment Satisfaction Questionnaire (DTSQ) plus a questionnaire to assess the degree to which treatment outcomes corresponded to patient expectations. One study[55] used qualitative interviews to assess QOL but did not use a specific measure.

We also identified two HRQL measures that have been developed specifically for patients with DR: the Retinopathy Treatment Satisfaction Questionnaire (RetTSQ), and the Retinopathy Dependent Quality of Life (RetDQoL) measure. The HRQL assessment tools are described in Table ES2.

ES2. Description of health-related quality of life assessment tools

Instrument	Administration	Domains Measured	Scoring
Generic HRQL assessment tools			
Short Form–36 (SF–36)	**Target population:** general pt population, aged >14 yr **Mode of administration:** self-complete questionnaire **Time needed to complete:** 5–10 minutes	Physical functioning; Role limitations because of physical health problems; Bodily pain; Social functioning; General mental health; Role limitations because of emotional problems; Vitality; General health perceptions; Health transition **Items:** 8 items (excluding health transition)	**Possible range:** 0 (least favorable) to 100 (most favorable)
Low-vision HRQL assessment tools			
National Eye Institute Visual Function Questionnaire–25 (VFQ–25)	**Target population:** pt with low vision **Mode of administration:** pt interview; self-administered **Time needed to complete:** 5 minutes	Overall health; Overall vision; Difficulty with: i) near vision; ii) distance vision; Limitations in social functioning; Role limitations; Dependency on others; Mental health symptoms; Driving difficulties; Pain and discomfort around the eyes; Peripheral vision; Color vision **Items:** 25 or 26 items (versions vary between 2 and 3 questions in the driving domain)	**Possible range:** 0 (most severe impairment) to 100 (no impairment)
Visual Function–14 (VF–14)	**Target population:** pt treated with cataract surgery **Mode of administration:** NR **Time needed to complete:** NR	Vision dependent functional activities: e.g. reading; recognizing people; seeing steps, stairs or curbs; doing fine handwork; writing checks or filling out forms; playing games, taking part in sports, cooking, watching television; and driving **Items:** 18 questions cover 14 items	**Possible range:** 0 (most severe impairment) to100 (no impairment)

DM = diabetes mellitus; DR = diabetic retinopathy; NR = not reported; pt = patient; QOL = quality of life tx = treatment; yr = year

ES2. Description of health-related quality of life assessment tools (continued)

Instrument	Administration	Domains Measured	Scoring
Diabetes-related HRQL assessment tools			
Diabetes Treatment Satisfaction Questionnaire Status Version (DTSQs)	**Target population:** pt with DM **Mode of administration:** self-completed questionnaire **Time needed to complete:** NR	Treatment Satisfaction; Perceived frequency of hyperglycemia; Perceived frequency of hypoglycemia **Items:** 8 items	**Possible range:** *Treatment Satisfaction:* 0 (most dissatisfied) to 36 (most satisfied); *Perceived frequency of hyperglycemia/hypoglycemia:* 0 (least frequent) to 6 (most frequent)
Diabetic retinopathy-related HRQL assessment tools			
Retinopathy Dependent Quality of Life (RetDQoL)	**Target population:** pt with DR **Mode of administration:** paper based questionnaire **Time needed to complete:** NR	Retinopathy-dependent quality of life: e.g. household tasks; personal affairs; shopping; feelings about the future/past; working life; close personal relationship; family life; social life **Items:** 24 items, also assesses the importance of each item to the pt	**Possible range:** -9 (max negative impact of DR on QOL) to 3 (max positive impact of DR on QOL)
Retinopathy Treatment Satisfaction Questionnaire (RetTSQ)	**Target population** pt with DR **Mode of administration:** paper based questionnaire **Time needed to complete:** NR	Satisfaction of treatment for DR: e.g. tx satisfaction, perceived effectiveness of tx; tx side effects; discomfort or pain; unpleasantness of tx; difficulty of tx; feelings of apprehension r/t tx; feelings of satisfaction regarding influence over tx; safety of tx; time-consumed by tx; **Items:** 13 items asking pt to rate different aspects of treatment	**Possible range:** *0* (worst) to 78 (best)

DM = diabetes mellitus; DR = diabetic retinopathy; NR = not reported; pt = patient; QOL = quality of life tx = treatment; yr = year

Key Question 1b. What are the psychometric properties of the HRQL measures used in the studies?

The six HRQL tools can be separated into two broad groups: generic and specific. The latter category can be further divided into tools developed for use in populations with low vision, diabetes mellitus, and DR. Table ES3 presents a summary of the ratings of the psychometric properties for the measurement tools.

ES3. Rating of the psychometric properties of health-related quality of life assessment tools used in studies of treatment of diabetic retinopathy

Measure	Content validity	Construct validity	Internal consistency	Test re-test reliability	Measurement error	Responsiveness	Interpretability
SF-36	+	+	+	+	+	+	+
VFQ-25	+	+	+	+	0	?	?
VF-14	?	+	+	?	0	?	0
DTSQ	+	+	+	+	+	+	0
RetDQoL	+	+	+	0	0	0	0
RetTSQ	+	+	+	0	0	0	0

Method or result was rated as: + = high quality; ? = indeterminate; - = low quality; 0 = no data available

Key Questions 2 and 3: What is the evidence that HRQL is improved by any intervention; and what is the relationship between HRQL and any relevant variables?

We identified two RCTs[42,47] and seven observational studies that addressed Key Questions 2 and 3. Sample sizes ranged from 55 to 345 (IQR: 77 – 293.5). Both RCTs were multicenter trials that recruited patients in Australia, North and South America, Europe, India and Turkey. Both trials were assessed as having unclear risk of bias. The primary concern was incomplete reporting and the use of the last observation carried forward approach for missing data. Both trials received industry funding.

For the observational studies, the interventions included laser photocoagulation,[48,54] vitrectomy,[41,45,46] panretinal photocoagulation,[46] and phacoemulsification cataract surgery for diabetic patients with cataracts.[51,53] Two of the four cohort studies were of good quality, and all three before-after studies were of moderate to good quality. However, overall this collection of observational studies is at high risk of bias due to weak study designs (before-after and cohort studies). We conducted a post hoc analysis of the subgroup of patients with diabetic macular edema (DME). Six studies[41,42,45,47,48,54] reported results for those with DME. Two studies[51,53] included patients with DME, but did not report separate results. Patients with DME represented less than five percent of the study sample in these studies. One study[46] did not report whether patients with DME were included in their study.

Results

Anti-Vascular Endothelial Growth Factor (anti-VEGF). Two RCTs provided data (Table ES4). One RCT reported data on the administration of pegaptanib sodium versus sham injections—133 patients received 0.3 mg of pegaptanib sodium and 127 patients received a sham treatment. All patients were diagnosed with DME. The patients receiving pegaptanib sodium reported statistically significant improvements from baseline on the VFQ–25 domains for near vision activities, distance vision activities, and social functioning at 54 weeks compared with patients treated with a sham injection. There were no statistically significant differences for the other domains or for the composite score. At 102 weeks patients receiving pegaptanib sodium reported statistically significant improvements in the composite score and the domains for distance vision activities, social functioning, and mental health. One three-arm RCT reported data on the administration of ranibizumab with and without laser treatment—116 patients received 0.5 mg of ranibizumab plus sham laser, 118 patients received 0.5 mg of ranibizumab plus laser, and 111 patients received sham treatment plus laser. All patients were diagnosed with DME. The composite score and the scores on the domains for general vision, near vision activities, and distance activities of the VFQ–25 were significantly improved from baseline to 12 months for patients treated with ranibizumab alone, or in combination with laser treatment compared with patients with laser treatment only. The strength of evidence for anti-VEGF is low. Further research is likely to change the confidence in the estimate of effect and is likely to change the estimate.

Laser photocoagulation. Two before-after studies provided data (Table ES4). In one study, 105 patients with PDR and DME reported high scores on the DTSQ at 9 months following surgery. Results were not reported separately for the two groups of patients. In the second study, 55 patients with DME reported a statistically significant improvement in HRQL at 3 months following surgery. While HRQL improved following laser photocoagulation, the strength of evidence is insufficient to draw conclusions about the effect of laser photocoagulation on HRQL.

Vitrectomy. One cohort study and one before-after study provided data (Table ES4). In the prospective cohort study, 99 patients with PDR reported a statistically significant improvement on the VFQ–25 (Japanese version) at 3 months following surgery. For those with DME (n = 38), the score improved, but the change was not statistically significant. The score on the VFQ–25 for the normal control group was statiscally significantly higher than the preoperative and postoperative scores of patients with PDR and DME.

In the before-after study, 41 patients with vitreous hemorrhage reported statistically significant improvements on the VFQ–25 (Japanese version) at 6 months following surgery. This contrasts with patients with DME (n = 28) who reported no significant change in HRQL and fibrovascular membrane (n = 18) who only reported a statistically significant change on the general vision subscale. While HRQL improved for some subgroups of patients with DR following vitrectomy, the strength of evidence is insufficient to draw conclusions about the effect of vitrectomy on HRQL.

Vitrectomy and panretinal photocoagulation. One cohort study (Table ES4) provided data for 327 patients with DR. Of these, 136 underwent vitrectomy, 60 received panretinal photocoagulation, and 131 had no treatment and served as a comparison group. For the vitrectomy group, there was a statistically significant improvement in the VFQ–25 (Japanese version) composite score at 1 year following surgery. Changes in the VFQ–25 scores for the comparison group and the photocoagulation group were not statistically significant. The strength of evidence is insufficient to draw conclusions about the relative effect of vitrectomy versus panretinal photocoagulation on HRQL.

Phacoemulsifcation. Two cohort studies provided data (Table ES4). One study evaluated visual outcomes and visual function using the VF–14 after first-eye phacoemulsification cataract surgery. Three months following surgery, 94 percent of patients reported improved visual acuity, and 93 percent reported improvements in visual function. Patients with no DR or mild retinopathy demonstrated significantly greater improvements in visual acuity and visual function compared with patients with more advanced DR.

The second study followed 89 diabetic patients with bilateral cataracts. At 12 months following surgery, patients with PDR had the lowest VF–14 scores at baseline and improved marginally over the study period regardless of whether they had cataract surgery on one or both eyes. A similar pattern was seen for patients with moderate or severe NPDR. For patients with no or mild NPDR, maximum VF–14 scores at 12 months were significantly higher than for patients with more severe DR.

The impact of first-eye cataract surgery on QOL was evident in patients with no or mild DR with the highest VF–14 scores being achieved by 91 percent of patients in the first month. In contrast, for those with more severe DR, 79 percent achieved the highest VF–14 score after 3 months. In patients with no or mild DR who underwent second-eye surgery the improved functional status achieved after first surgery was sustained. For those who did not have second-eye surgery, VF–14 scores decreased after 8 and 12 months. While HRQL improved following phacoemulsification cataract surgery, the strength of evidence is insufficient to draw conclusions about the effect of this surgery on HRQL.

Factors associated with outcomes. No conclusions can be drawn about factors associated with HRQL outcomes. In one study, multivariate analysis found that age <65 years, more severe level of DR, and low preoperative QOL were associated with improved HRQL following laser photocoagulation. In another study that also investigated laser photocoagulation, univariate analysis showed an association between age and treatment satisfaction, with older patients (>65 years) being more satisfied.

In a study that looked at vitrectomy, multivariate analysis showed that improvement in contrast sensitivity was significantly correlated with changes in the VFQ–25 composite score for patients with PDR and DME. There was no significant correlation between VFQ–25 and visual acuity.

Discussion

Using a comprehensive search strategy and concerted efforts to avoid publication and selection bias, this review identified the evidence on the effect that interventions for DR, including DME have on HRQL. Overall we identified four measures—one generic, two vision-specific, and one diabetes-specific—that have been used to measure HRQL in studies of treatment for DR. As well, we identified two recently developed tools that are specific to patients with DR. We identified two RCTs and seven observational studies involving between 55 and 345 patients that addressed the question of whether HRQL is improved for any intervention for DR.

HRQL Measures

Only one generic HRQL measure has been used to assess the impact that interventions for DR have on HRQL. The SF–36 gathers information about the patient's perceived health and asks about eight health concepts: physical functioning, physical role functioning, bodily pain, general health, vitality, social function, emotional role functioning, and mental health. Generic HRQL tools are generally insensitive to the presence of specific eye disease. Furthermore, the SF–36 appears to be unresponsive to changes in visual acuity in patients with DR.[49] The authors suggest that this may be because the SF–36 assesses a wide range of characteristics that are not directly related to visual acuity. While the SF–36 is a reasonable choice for researchers to consider if a generic health status measure is needed, other generic measures that include assessment of vision function (e.g., the Health Utilities Index[76]) may be worth consideration for this patient population. Generic HRQL tools can be used to make comparisons with the general population (regardless of the underlying condition), and to estimate the relative impact of various medical conditions.[20,23,49] The decision to use a generic measure along with a specific measure needs to be driven by the purpose of the measurement.[35]

Two validated and clinically responsive vision-specific measures, the VFQ–25 and VF–14, have been used to measure the impact of different interventions on HRQL in individuals with DR. Vision-specific measures have been shown to be sensitive to differences in vision status and functioning among patients with DR.[50,63,64,66]

The diabetes-specific tool, the DTSQ, was specifically developed to measure satisfaction with treatment regimens in individuals with diabetes. Research has shown that satisfaction with treatment is associated with compliance with treatment.[77,78] The DTSQ was not designed to measure satisfaction with other aspects of the diabetes care and management.[67] It is most useful when used as one of a profile of tools to assess other important outcomes, including QOL or HRQL.

We identified two disease-specific measures developed specifically for patients with DR – the RetDQoL and the RetTSQ. The tools have been developed in parallel, and to date, are the only measures that assess the impact of DR on different aspects of QOL. Unlike other tools identified in this review, the RetDQoL and RetTSQ have been designed to enable patients to consider specifically the impact of diabetic eye problems and their treatment, rather than health generally, vision or vision loss, or impact of diabetes.[18] Preliminary psychometric testing appears promising for content validity and internal consistency. Additional testing is ongoing to assess test-retest reliability, responsiveness, and interpretability.

Despite the availability of reliable and valid tools to measure HRQL,[20,28,35] our review identified several studies that used questions or tools whose psychometric properties have not been evaluated. In order to provide meaningful HRQL data, it is crucial that the measurement tools are reliable, valid, and responsive (i.e., sensitive to change). In this way, researchers, clinicians, and patients will be better able to assess and interpret the impact of different interventions on HRQL outcomes.

Impact of interventions on HRQL

To date, two RCTs have reported HRQL outcomes.[42,47] More are expected as a search of Clinicaltrails.gov identified 13 ongoing or recently completed trials investigating interventions for DME or DR that indicate the intention to report HRQL outcomes. The PKC-DRS2 trial of once-daily ruboxistaurin versus placebo measured HRQL using the SF–36 and the VFQ–25;[75] however, results for the HRQL outcomes have not been reported. Futhermore, preliminary results from the RISE and RIDE trials[79] comparing ranibizumab versus sham have been presented at national meetings; however, to date, the final results for HRQL have not been published.

In general, it appears that HRQL outcomes improve following various interventions to treat DR at different levels of severity. For anti-VEGF to treat patients with DME, two RCTs with unclear risk of bias found statistically significant improvements in some domains of the VFQ–

25; however, the results were not consistent at 1 year post-treatment. We concluded that the strength of evidence was low.

For other interventions, the results are based on one or two observational studies with a high risk of bias. Therefore, we conclude that the strength of evidence is insufficient to draw any conclusions about which of these interventions for DR are effective in improving HRQL. Furthermore, there is a concern about the applicability of the results of the observational studies to patients in North America. All of these studies were conducted in Europe or Japan. In particular, the three studies that were based in Japan used the Japanese version of the VFQ–25.

This review shows that the impact of interventions for DR on HRQL has not been adequately assessed in the current literature. Research has increasingly highlighted HRQL as an important health outcome in diabetes.[35] Diabetic patients with retinopathy have reported that vision loss impacts multiple areas of well-being including: independence, mobility, leisure, and self-care.[7,17,18] However, the impact of DR is due not only to impaired vision, but also the emotional reaction to diagnosis and treatment, anxiety about the future, and advice to restrict physical activities.[18] For researchers and clinicians conducting trials of interventions for DR, the inclusion of HRQL outcomes will provide a better understanding how DR and its treatment affects outcomes that are important to patients.

Table ES4. Study characteristics and outcomes for studies reporting the impact of interventions for diabetic retinopathy on HRQL

Author Year Study design Country	Intervention HRQL measure Followup	Participants	Visual acuity outcomes	HRQL outcomes
Anti-VEGF				
Mitchell 2011[47] RCT Multicenter (73 centers in Australia, Canada, Europe, Turkey)	G1—ranibizumab 0.5 mg + sham laser G2—ranibizumab 0.5 mg + laser G3—laser + sham injection VFQ-25 3 mo, 12 mo	G1 = 116 G2 = 118 G3 = 111 DME = 345 (100%)	Median change in BCVA from baseline to 12 mo: G1 = 6.1±6.43 G2 = 5.9±7.92 G3 = 0.8±8.59 Median change in BCVA from baseline to 12 mo: G1 = 6.1 (-10.9–25.2) G2 = 6.0 (-26.7–27.6) G3 = 1.3 (-37.8–26.8) 95% CI for the mean change: G1 = 4.9, 7.3 G2 = 4.4, 7.3 G3 = -0.8, 2.4	VFQ-25, composite score at 12 mo G1—baseline: NR; improvement: 5.0 (p=0.014 compared to G3) G2—baseline: NR; improvement: 5.4 (p=0.004 compared to G3)) G3—baseline: NR; improvement: 0.6 (NR) Other domains: G1—significant improvement for general vision, near vision activities, distance activities; other domains: NR G2— significant improvement for general vision, near vision activities, distance activities; other domains: NR G3—baseline: NR; no significant change from baseline
Sultan 2011[42] RCT Multicenter (60 centers in Australia, Europe, India, North America, South America)	G1—pegaptanib 0.3 mg G2—sham injection VFQ-25 baseline, 18, 54 & 102 wk	G1 = 133 G2 = 127 DME = 260 (100%)	% improvement of ≥10 letters from baseline at 54 wk: G1 = 43/133 (36.8%) G2 = 25/127 (19.7%) Odds ratio (95% CI) = 2.38 (1.32, 4.30); p=0.0047 % improvement of ≥10 letters from baseline at 102 wk G1 = 41/107 (38.3%) G2 = 30/100 (30%) Odds ratio (95% CI) = 1.57 (0.83, 2.97); p=0.1729	VFQ-25, composite score at 54 wk: G1—70.4; improvement 4.5 G2—69.2; improvement 1.3 Between group differences—2.92; range -0.32 to 6.16 (p = 0.077) VFQ-25, composite score at 102 wk (n = 207): G1—69.8; improvement 4.6 G2—66.2; improvement 0.1 Between group differences—4.47; range -0.26 to 8.68 (p = 0.038) Other domains: 54 wk: G1 vs. G2 had significantly more improvement for near vision activities, distance activities, social functioning; no difference for other domains 102 wk: G1 vs. G2 had significantly more improvement for distance activities, social functioning, mental health; no difference for other domains

95% CI = 95 percent confidence interval; BCVA = best corrected visual acuity; DR = diabetic retinopathy; DTSQ = Diabetes Treatment Satisfaction Questionnaire; DME = diabetic macular edema; mg = milligram; mo = month; NPDR = nonproliferative diabetic retinopathy; PDR = proliferative diabetic retinopathy; VF–14 = Visual Function–14; VFQ = National Eye Institute Visual Function Questionnaire; wk = week; yr = year

Table ES4. Study characteristics and outcomes for studies reporting the impact of interventions for diabetic retinopathy on HRQL (continued)

Author Year Study design Country	Intervention HRQL measure Followup	Participants	Visual acuity outcomes	HRQL outcomes
Laser photocoagulation				
Tranos 2004[48] Before-after United Kingdom	Laser photocoagulation VFQ–51 3 mo	DME = 55 (100%) Mild NPDR = 13 Moderate NPDR = 32 Severe NPDR = 10	Binocular vision—baseline: 48.7±6.7 Distance vision—baseline: 42.7±8.4 letters; improvement: 2.2±6.2 Near vision—baseline: 56.4±9.1 letters; improvement: 2.1±5.0	Composite score—baseline: 77.9±17.6; improvement: 4.9±8.9 ($p<0.001$); Subscales—statistically significant improvement on 8 of 11 vision-related domains
Mozaffarieh 2005b[54] Before-after Austria	Laser photocoagulation DTSQ 9 mo	Total = 105 PDR = 56 (53%) DME = 49 (47%)	24.7% reported improvement in visual acuity; 71.4% were unchanged; 3.8% were worse No difference in improvement between patients with PDR or DME	Mean± SD = 27.9±5.2 (maximum possible score = 36)
Vitrectomy				
Emi 2008[45] Before-after Japan	Vitrectomy VFQ–25 (Japanese version) 6 mo	DR = 87 (total) G1—vitreous hemorrhage = 41 G2—DME = 28 G3—fibrovascular membrane = 18	G1—improved: 35; unchanged: 4; worse: 2 G2—improved: 9; unchanged: 16; worse: 3 G3—improved: 13; unchanged: 3; worse: 2	G1—statistically significant improvement on 10 of 12 subscales G2—no statistically significant change from baseline on any subscales G3—only the general vision subscale had a statistically significant improvement from baseline
Okamoto 2010[41] Prospective cohort Japan	Pars plana vitrectomy VFQ–25 (Japanese version) 3 mo	G1—PDR = 99 G2—DME = 38 G3—normal controls = 100 Note: this is part of a larger study (n = 399) of patients with vitreoretinal disorders—retinal vein occlusion (32), macular hole (42), epiretinal membrane (33), retinal detachment (55)	logMAR G1—baseline: 1.37±0.75; 3 mo: 0.53±0.62 ($p < 0.0001$) G2—baseline = 0.76±0.49; 3 mo: 0.55±0.51 ($p < 0.01$) Contrast sensitivity G1—baseline: 5.4±7.2; 3 mo: 14.0±7.9 ($p < 0.0001$) G2—baseline 9.2±6.5; 3 mo: 12.7±7.1 ($p < 0.0001$)	G1—baseline: 52.8±19.0; 3 mo: 63.6±17.5 ($p <0.001$); Subscales—statistically significant improvement on 9/11 vision-related domains G2—baseline: 53.0±20.5; 3 mo: 59.0±21.0 (p = 0.84); Subscales—statistically significant improvement on 4/11 vision-related domains G3—85.0±9.1

Table ES4. Study characteristics and outcomes for studies reporting the impact of interventions for diabetic retinopathy on HRQL (continued)

Author Year Study design Country	Intervention HRQL measure Followup	Participants	Visual acuity outcomes	HRQL outcomes
Vitrectomy and panretinal photocoagulation				
Emi 2009[46] Prospective cohort Japan	G1—vitrectomy G2—panretinal photocoagulation G3—no treatment VFQ-25 (Japanese version) 1 yr	G1 = 136 G2 = 60 G3 = 131	*logMAR—right eye* G1—baseline: 0.21; 1 yr: 0.46 ($p < 0.001$) G2—baseline: 0.64; 1 yr: 0.52 ($p = 0.272$) G3—baseline: 1.09; 1 yr: 1.06 ($p = 0.294$) *logMAR—left eye* G1—baseline: 0.19; 1 yr: 0.38 ($p < 0.001$) G2—baseline: 0.61; 1 yr: 0.56 ($p = 0.081$) G3—baseline: 1.10; 1 yr: 1.09 ($p = 0.704$)	*Composite score* G1—baseline: 67.4±17.3; 1 yr: 75.4±17.5 ($p < 0.001$) G2—baseline: 80.7±15.7; 1 yr: 77.6±19.1 ($p = 0.113$) G3—baseline: 91.3±7.8; 1 yr: 92.2±7.8 ($p = 0.169$)
Phacoemulsification cataract surgery				
Mozaffarieh 2005a[53] Prospective cohort Austria	Phacoemulsification cataract surgery VF-14 3 mo	Cataracts = 67 (total) G1—no DR = 17 G2—mild NPDR = 19 G3—moderate/severe NPDR = 16 G4—PDR = 15	*logMAR (range)* G1—baseline: 0.62 (0.30–1.30); improvement 0.55 (0.30–1.15) G2—baseline: 0.60 (0.30–1.30); improvement 0.50 (0.30–1.08) G3—baseline: 0.67 (0.30–1.30); improvement 0.26 (0.15–0.48) G4—baseline: 0.71 (0.40–1.30); improvement 0.15 (-0.70–0.60)	G1—baseline: 52.21 (32.14–78.57); improvement 42.33 (21.43–60.71) G2—baseline: 55.92 (30.36–85.71); improvement 36.00 (12.50–58.93) G3—baseline: 46.65 (30.36–64.29); improvement 9.26 (1.79–25.00) G4—baseline: 40.12 (25.00–67.86); improvement 5.00 (-25.00–25.00)
Mozaffarieh 2009[51] Prospective cohort Austria	Phacoemulsification cataract surgery G1—first-eye surgery G2—both eyes VF-14 12 mo	Cataracts = 89 (total) No DR = 23 Mild NPDR = 23 Moderate NPDR = 22 PDR = 21	G1 & G2—patients with no or mild NPDR had greater improvement in visual acuity	G1 baseline: no DR: 59.3±12.4; mild 39.3±5.2; severe 40.9±8.6; PDR 35.3±4.4 6 mo: no DR: 96.8±2.0; mild 86.5±13.6; severe 48.8±6.7; PDR 37.9±14.0 12 mo: no DR: 79.5±5.5; mild 72.2±8.3; severe 46.1±10.7; PDR 39.9±9.0 G2 baseline: no DR 46.8±8.7; mild 63.4±16.3; severe 54.6±8.8; PDR 50.6±11.4 6 mo: no DR: 93.0±4.3; mild 94.6±2.5; severe 60.9±6.6; PDR 53.0±10.9 12 mo: no DR: 95.3±1.9; mild 95.3±2.2; severe 47.8±16.0; PDR 47.6±15.0

Recommendations for Future Research

- RCTs are needed to assess the impact of interventions for DR, including DME on HRQL. All RCTs investigating the effectiveness of interventions for DR should measure and report pre- and post-treatment HRQL outcomes.
- Currently, there are a number of ongoing or recently completed trials that reported the intention to capture HRQL outcomes. Future systematic reviews on this topic should followup on these studies and incorporate their findings, if appropriate.
- Researchers should use valid and reliable HRQL tools whose psychometric properties have been evaluated and reported.
- Ongoing assessment of the psychometric properties of the DR specific tools is encouraged.
- Patients should be followed for at least 6 months post-intervention in order to capture maximum improvement for visual acuity.
- Researchers should use standard protocols to assess visual acuity to allow for comparison across trials
- RCTs should be designed and conducted to minimize risk of bias where at all possible. Authors may find tools such as the CONSORT[18,76] statement helpful in designing and reporting on RCTs.

Conclusions

We identified four HRQL measurement instruments that have been used to assess the impact of treatment in patients with DR. The psychometric properties of these tools have been adequately evaluated. Two tools developed specifically for patients with DR are currently undergoing evaluation. In general, HRQL was improved following interventions for DR. Further research on HRQL following anti-VEGF treatment for DME is needed to confirm the results of two RCTs. The current research on the impact of other interventions for DR on HRQL is insufficient to draw conclusions about the relative effect of one intervention versus another. RCTs that assess the impact of treatments for DR should include HRQL as an outcome.

Introduction

The Coverage and Analysis Group at the Centers for Medicare and Medicaid Services (CMS) requested this report from the Technology Assessment Program (TAP) at the Agency for Healthcare Research and Quality (AHRQ). AHRQ assigned this report to the following Evidence-based Practice Center: University of Alberta Evidence-based Practice Center (Contract No. HHSA 290 2007 10021 I).

Diabetic Retinopathy

Diabetic retinopathy (DR) is a leading cause of vision loss in the United States and occurs as a result of pathologic changes of the retinal vasculature.[1] In 2005–2008, the estimated crude prevalence among Americans over the age of 40 with diabetes was 28.5 percent. Although the prevalence of vision-threatening DR is approximately 4.4 percent,[2] the number of affected Americans 40 years or older is expected to triple from 1.2 million in 2005 to 3.4 million in 2050.[3] The prevalence and severity of DR increases with the duration of diabetes; however, it is inversely correlated to glycemic and blood pressure control.[4,5] Moderate vision loss is most commonly related to retinal leakage within the macula, while severe vision loss usually occurs as a result of neovascularization (proliferative diabetic retinopathy; PDR) with subsequent hemorrhage or fibrosis.[6]

Early identification and treatment of DR is an important goal for patients and health systems because treatment is both cost-effective and reduces vision loss.[7] Therefore, early detection is critical; the American Academy of Ophthalmologists, the American Optometric Association, and the American Diabetes Association recommend an annual dilated eye examination for all people with diabetes, and more frequent eye examinations for people with known DR.[8-10] Other researchers argue that the frequency of examinations should be stratified to an individual's risk of progression and vision loss.[11]

The mainstay of DR treatment is aimed at reducing the risk of onset and limiting the progression of the disease. Therefore, retinal assessments should be performed on a regular basis to determine the presence and degree of DR, glycemic control should be optimized, and known risk factors such as blood pressure, dyslipidemia, elevated cholesterol, renal disease and abdominal obesity should be controlled. Direct ocular therapy should be prescribed when indicated, while vision rehabilitation and low vision aids should to be used to maximize vision if there is a loss.[4,5]

Until recently, the primary treatment for DR has been focal or grid laser of the retina.[12,13] Serial intravitreal injections of triamcinolone have been introduced as a treatment option as they have been shown to be effective in reducing diabetic macular edema (DME); however, their use has become less common due to significant adverse effects including elevated intraocular pressure and cataract formation.[14,15] Ranibizumab and becvacizumab are being used with increasing frequency for the treatment of DME; however they have not yet been approved for use in this condition by the Food and Drug Administration. The recommended treatment of PDR remains panretinal photocoagulation[16] with vitrectomy surgery performed when necessary.[14] It is important to note that treatment of DR is not always aimed at restoration of pre-disease visual acuity, but rather at limiting further deterioration. Patients may report a decrease in visual acuity immediately after therapy, which may manifest in low initial perceptions of treatment satisfaction. However, results from the Early Treatment Diabetic Retinopathy Study demonstrate that early treatment with either panretinal photocoagulation or vitrectomy prevents long-term disability due to blindness.[12-14]

Vision loss is particularly debilitating for patients with diabetes because treatment success to limit progression of their diabetes depends upon their ability to read a glucometer and inject subcutaneous insulin. Diabetic patients with retinopathy have reported that vision loss impacts multiple areas of well-being including: independence, mobility, leisure, and self-care.[7,17,18] Additionally, DR has been found to impair functioning and overall health-related quality of life (HRQL).[19,20]

Health-Related Quality of Life

Patient-Reported Outcomes

In recent years clinicians and researchers have given greater recognition to the subjective experiences of patients diagnosed with chronic illnesses such as diabetes mellitus. This increase in attention targets a more holistic understanding of the patient and how treatments purported to curtail long-term complications of chronic illnesses, such as DR, affect daily physical and psychosocial functioning.[21] Patient reported outcomes (PROs) are a group of outcomes used to measure a wide variety of aspects of care including HRQL, patient illness perceptions, and treatment satisfaction or adherence.[21] PROs can be distinguished from other outcomes such as laboratory results and clinician or caregiver ratings because the report is from the patient's perspective, usually without interpretation by another individual.[22] Furthermore, PROs are dependent on disease-related dimensions, such as the degree of visual impairment caused by DR.[21] Researchers are more frequently including PROs as a part of clinical trials as they help demonstrate benefit, survival, and patient feelings regarding treatments.[22] However, PROs tend to be evaluated as a secondary outcome, and are rarely the primary outcome of a trial.[21]

Health Status/Functional Status

Included under the umbrella of PROs are the terms: health status, functional status, and quality of life (QOL) or HRQL. These terms are frequently used interchangeably to mean "health"; however, researchers caution that they have distinct meanings and uses.[23,24] Health status is often used to refer to the identification and assessment of changes in patients' activities and perceptions compared with normal life.[24] This construct is multidimensional and represents patients' subjective evaluations of their physical and mental health.[25] Functional status focuses on the physical capacity to complete everyday activities at home or work, rather than patients' perceptions of how their health affects their functioning.[25] Health status is effective in monitoring the status of a community or local population and can be used in setting health priorities, identifying high risk groups, estimating service needs, and analyzing usage patterns.[24] HRQL and QOL delve further into patient perceptions of health and well-being.

Health-Related Quality of Life/Quality of Life

QOL covers a range of experiences related to patients' well-being based on their subjective experiences.[25] Many variables, both objective and subjective, interact to define QOL,[26] but it is dependent upon individual patient experiences, states, and perceptions of their illness.[25] QOL can vary as a result of life events or changes in functional health status, with each area of QOL impacting the others.[26] In the case of patients with diabetes, comorbidities and complications such as renal disease or dialysis, neuropathy, gastroparesis, amputation, impotence and erectile dysfunction all play a part in influencing QOL. Furthermore, the level of visual acuity, glycemic control, and duration of disease can impact directly on vision-related QOL.

HRQL allows clinicians and researchers to measure the impact of chronic diseases such as diabetes mellitus on the lives of patients.[23] As with QOL, HRQL is a multifaceted measurement. It takes into account the impact of disease and its treatments on physical, psychological, social, and somatic domains of functioning and well-being.[25] Therefore, in patients diagnosed with DR, treatments that improve visual acuity also have the potential to positively impact HRQL by allowing them to continue participating, or to increase their ability to participate, in the daily activities of their lives. Various domains can be included in the evaluation of HRQL including physical, psychological, and social assessments. Some definitions may include broader terms such as global perceptions of functioning and general well-being.[25] Several different views exist on how to measure QOL and HRQL, in large part due their subjective nature, but also due to the lack of distinction between indicator and causal variables, as well as mediating variables.[26]

Measuring Health-Related Quality of Life/Quality of Life

As patient-centered health care grows in importance, clinicians and researchers need a way to make health care decisions that meet the needs of patients. It is critical to ensure that treatment decisions meet patient and societal values, and to recognize that perceptions of HRQL may vary between the patient and clinicians.[25] Furthermore, investigations into public perceptions of HRQL and QOL suggest that areas judged important by the general public have not been included in some commonly used measurement tools.[26] Collecting HRQL and QOL outcomes allows clinicians and researchers to take into account a wider array of information that cannot be obtained through laboratory or physical measures, and permit a subjective description of functioning alongside objective findings.[27] Through the collection of patient perceptions of interventions used to treat DR, health care providers can better understand what aspects of health patients value most highly and therefore what types of treatment may provide the greatest benefit.

Just as the definitions of HRQL and QOL vary, so too do the tools used for evaluating these outcomes. Evaluation tools may be as simple as a single question asking the patient to state their QOL; however, they are more likely to take the form of a questionnaire with multiple items, which investigate different domains related to HRQL.[23] The common thread that exists among measurement tools is that they attempt to summarize the judgments patients make about their health and illness experiences.[26] HRQL tools can be placed into two categories: generic instruments- and specific instruments.

Generic HRQL tools investigate all important aspects of HRQL and allow broad comparisons, but do not necessarily investigate a specific aspect of disease. Typically generic tools include questions relating to the four main domains of HRQL: physical, functional, social, and psychological health.[28] These tools may be less responsive to change as they provide an overall summary score of HRQL, rather than a score on a precise area of health.[23] Of the tools investigated in this review, one falls into the category of generic tools. The Short Form–36 (SF–36) questionnaire investigates eight health domains in patients with a variety of conditions and was developed for use in the general patient population.

Specific HRQL instruments are designed to target a disease, population, or an outcome. Where generic tools allow broad comparisons, specific tools may be more responsive to HRQL changes in the specific patient population under investigation.[23] Two tools included in this review were developed specifically to evaluate patients with eye disease: the Visual Function–14 (VF–14), and the National Eye Institute Visual Function Questionnaire (VFQ) (both 25 and 51 item versions). These tools were designed for patients diagnosed with cataracts and low vision, respectively, but do not investigate the involvement of the underlying condition of diabetes mellitus on patient QOL. One tool included in this review, the Diabetic Treatment Satisfaction Questionnaire (DTSQ), evaluates treatment satisfaction in patients with diabetes mellitus. This measure is disease-specific but it does not take into account whether or not a patient is also diagnosed with DR. Two tools included in this review were developed to evaluate HRQL in patients with DR: the Retinopathy Treatment Satisfaction Questionnaire (RetTSQ), and the Retinopathy Dependent Quality of Life (RetDQoL) questionnaire. Since diabetic patients without retinopathy may have different concerns compared to those with retinopathy, these tools have the potential to provide a greater understanding of HRQL than a tool such as the DTSQ. Both of these tools have undergone a series of psychometric evaluations; however, to date neither has been used in published trials assessing the impact of an intervention for DR.

Psychometric Properties for HRQL Tools

Regardless of whether a tool is generic or specific, it is helpful to accumulate evidence of its psychometric properties to ensure they provide the most reliable and valid assessment of health status in the patient population. Accompanying the growing interest in HRQL has been the increase in the number of tools available to measure such outcomes, which in turn can make it difficult for researchers and clinicians to determine what tools are the most trustworthy and appropriate for use in clinical and research settings. In recent years, researchers have undertaken the challenge of identifying what psychometric properties are of greatest importance when evaluating the quality of a HRQL tool, and what criteria should be used in judging the psychometric properties. In 2010 the COnsensus-based Standards for the selection of health Measurement INstruments (COSMIN) was released as a checklist for the purpose of evaluating the methodological quality of studies investigating the measurement properties of HRQL tools.[29] The COSMIN researchers used a Delphi approach to reach consensus on what psychometric properties are considered the most important for high-quality HRQL measurement instruments. They also reached consensus on definitions for these psychometric properties.

Reliability. Reliability is the degree to which the tool is free from measurement error.[29] Depending on the source of measurement error and how the measurement is obtained, reliability can take different forms. Internal consistency is a reflection of the reproducibility of measurement by different items within a multi-item scale. Test-retest reliability is the degree to which the score of a patient who has not changed clinically remains the same under repeated measurements;[29] other groups refer to this as reproducibility.[23,28,30] In order to ascertain test-retest reliability, measurements should be taken over an interval that is short enough to ensure that patients remain stable, but long enough to prevent recall bias. An interval of one to four weeks is considered sufficient.[23] Internal consistency reliability is commonly assessed using Cronbach's coefficient α. Test-retest reliability is typically presented as a correlation coefficient between the two sets of measurements, either Pearson's R or intra-class correlation. The minimum standard inter-item correlation for multi-item scales, for either reliability coefficient, is 0.70 for group comparisons, and 0.90 to 0.95 for individual comparisons.[30]

Validity. Validity is defined as the degree to which an instrument measures the construct(s) it is intended to measure.[29] The COSMIN panel identified three categories of validity: content validity, construct validity, and criterion validity. Content validity is concerned with the content of the measurement tool and whether it is an adequate reflection of the construct to be measured. Face validity is considered a part of this domain.[29] Typically, there are no formal tests of content validity, but rather a subjective assessment, based in part on the item generation process during instrument development. Construct validity considers whether the scores produced by the instrument are consistent with the hypothesis of how the tool should behave, assuming the tool is valid.[29] Achieving construct validity is often an iterative process.[31] Construct validity is further broken down into structural validity, hypothesis testing, and cross-cultural validity. The final type of validity, criterion validity, focuses on the degree to which the scores of an instrument reflect a "gold standard." Validity can be stronger when an instrument's results are tested against other known instruments;[30] however, the existence of gold standards in HRQL measurement tools is limited, therefore researchers may have to find alternate methods of demonstrating criterion validity.[23]

Responsiveness. The responsiveness of a tool demonstrates the ability of the instrument to detect changes in a patient over time when changes in the construct being measured actually occur.[29] Responsiveness, or a tool's sensitivity to change, is considered a specific type of construct validation when assessing change over time.[30] Hypotheses regarding the relationship of the change in the instrument and how they correspond to changes in reference measures should be proposed and tested.[28] Changes in HRQL measures can be compared with changes in a patient's health status, health events, interventions, or direct reports of change in QOL by patients or providers to help pinpoint the cause of variations in HRQL status.

Interpretability. The final domain considered by the COSMIN panel is interpretability. Interpretability is not seen as a psychometric property; rather it is important to assess the usability of the measurement tool. This domain is defined as the degree to which a clinician or researcher can equate a qualitative meaning to an instrument's quantitative score.[29] In other words, interpretability is concerned with whether or not an instrument can easily be understood and be made meaningful to clinicians and their patients.[30] Furthermore, interpretability is concerned with whether or not the score indicates that a patient is functioning normally, is experiencing moderate to severe impairment, or whether changes associated with treatments are small, medium or large.[23]

Key Questions

The Centers for Medicare and Medicaid Services (CMS) requested a technology assessment on the effectiveness of interventions for DR to improve HRQL. Four questions were posed:

1a. What HRQL measures have been used in studies of treatments for DR?
1b. What are the psychometric properties of the HRQL measures used in the studies?
2. Including only studies that have used reliable and valid measures, what is the evidence that HRQL is improved for any intervention for DR? What is the comparative effectiveness of interventions to improve HRQL in patients with DR?
3. What evidence is presented in the studies about the relationship between the measured improvement in HRQL and any relevant variables, including but not limited to baseline visual

acuity, age (≥ 65 years), race, sex, severity and type of DR (i.e. DME, nonproliferative diabetic retinopathy (NPDR), PDR)?

Analytic Framework

Figure 1 depicts the four key questions and the linkages between the population of interest, the interventions, and outcome measures. It demonstrates the chain of logic that the evidence obtained must support the link between the interventions, modifying variables, and patient outcomes. This technology assessment focuses primarily on the effect of interventions for DR on HRQL (Q2). HRQL instruments may differ in their psychometric properties, and these differences could be a source of variation in outcomes among studies that use different instruments (Q1a and Q1b). HRQL outcomes may be modified by demographic and clinical factors due to the variation in baseline prevalence of these factors in different populations (Q3). The specific HRQL instruments that have been used in studies and their psychometric properties will be reported separately from the patient outcomes.

Figure 1. Analytic Framework.

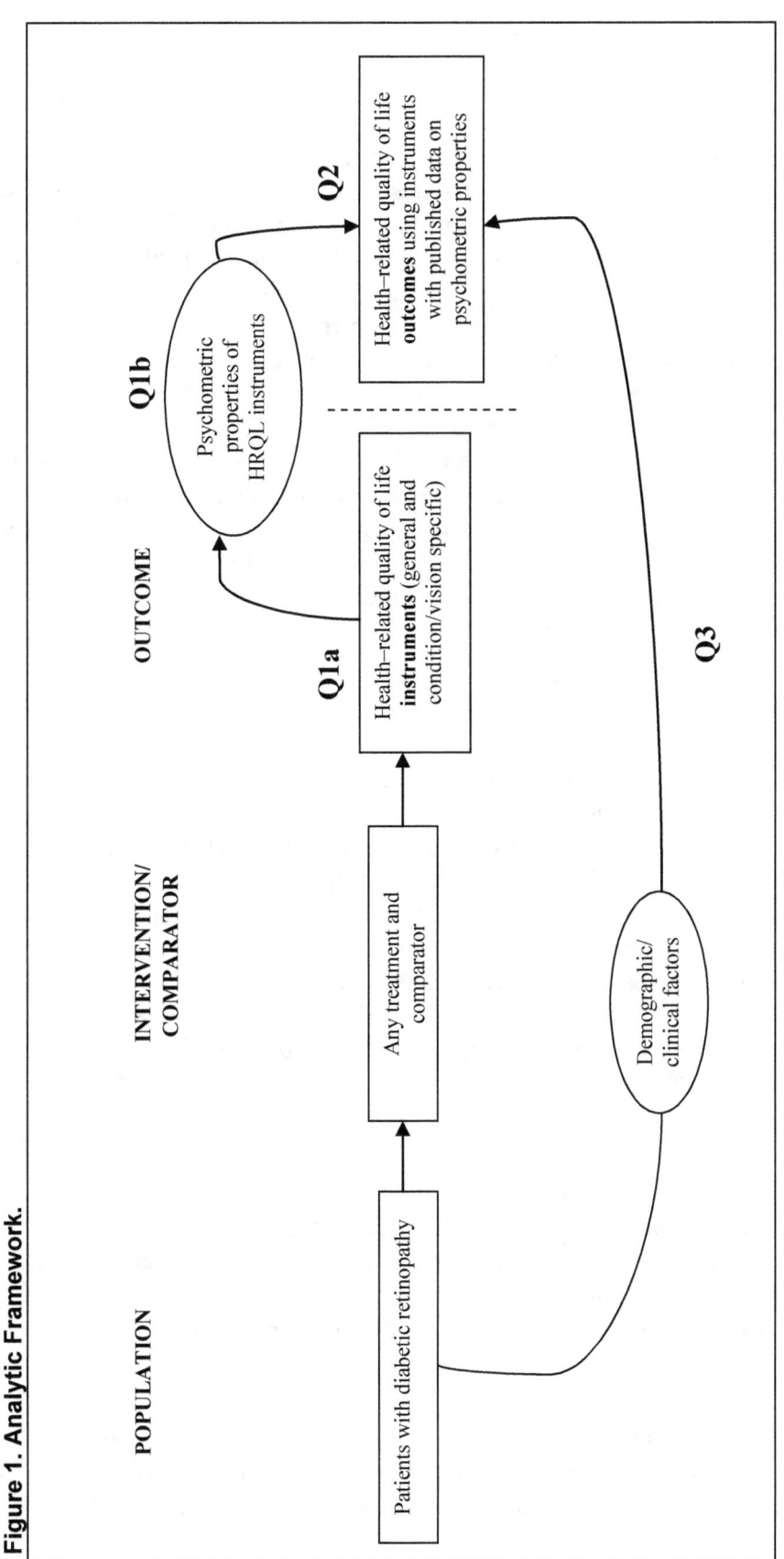

Methods

Literature Search

In consultation with a research librarian we conducted a comprehensive search of the literature to identify relevant studies to answer the Key Questions. A single search strategy was developed to locate literature to address all four questions and was run in July 2010 in the following databases: MEDLINE®, EMBASE®, PsychINFO®, Cochrane Central Register of Controlled Trials®, CINAHL Plus full text, and Scopus. The search was updated in March 2011 in MEDLINE®, EMBASE®, Cochrane Central Register of Controlled Trials®. PubMed was also searched at this time to ensure that all current literature was captured. A final updated search of all databases was conducted in January 2012. No date or language restrictions were applied. In all databases both subject headings and key word terms for "diabetes," "diabetic retinopathy," "quality of life," and "health-related quality of life" were included in the search. Appendix A contains a detailed description of the search strategy. We also conducted a search of clinicaltrials.gov for recently completed or ongoing studies of interest. The search was run in November 2010 then updated in April 2011 and used "diabetic retinopathy" as the main search term. The search was limited by study type (interventional studies) in adult participants.

To supplement the database searches we hand searched the reference lists of included studies and recently published review articles.[20,32-35]

Study Selection

We used a two-step process for study selection. First, three reviewers (AM, ES, KR) independently screened the titles and abstracts (when available) located through the literature search to determine if an article met broad inclusion criteria. Studies were classed as "include," "exclude," or "unsure." We retrieved the full-text of studies identified as "include," or "unsure," by at least one reviewer. Second, two reviewers (AM, KR) independently assessed each study using a standard inclusion-exclusion form (Appendix B). Disagreements were resolved through discussion between reviewers, or third party adjudication, as needed.

Our inclusion criteria are described below. Only articles published in full were considered for inclusion in this review (i.e., conference abstracts were not considered). We did not exclude studies based on their language of publication.

Study Design

For Key Question 1a and b all study designs were included.

For Key Questions 2 and 3, only prospective study designs with a comparator (i.e., randomized controlled trials (RCT), nonrandomized controlled trials (NRCT), quasi-experimental studies—including, but not limited to, controlled before-after studies—and prospective cohort studies) were included. Retrospective studies were excluded.

Population

For all questions, we included studies that recruited adults (≥18 years) who had been diagnosed with diabetic retinopathy (DR) including diabetic macular edema (DME), nonproliferative diabetic retinopathy (NPDR), proliferative diabetic retinopathy (PDR), and other related conditions.

Intervention and comparator

For all questions, we considered any intervention and comparator including comparisons of different types of interventions, different doses, or different formulations.

Outcome

For Key Questions 1a and 1b, any measurement instrument that included at least one domain of HRQL (i.e., physical, mental, emotional, social functioning) was considered.

For Key Questions 2 and 3, only outcomes based on measurement instruments with published data on the instrument's psychometric properties were included.

Data Extraction

Data were abstracted directly into evidence tables in a Microsoft Word™ document (Microsoft Corp., Redmond, WA). One reviewer abstracted data which was then checked for accuracy and completeness by a second reviewer. Disagreements were resolved through discussion or third party adjudication, as needed. The following data were extracted for Key Questions 1a and 1b: title of HRQL instrument, author(s), year of publication, instrument characteristics (target population, QOL domains measured, number of items, number of response options, scoring algorithm, time needed to complete, and mode of administration), and quality assessment for measurement properties.

The following data were extracted for Key Questions 2 and 3: author(s), year of publication, date of study, study setting, study characteristics (study design, inclusion/exclusion criteria, intervention, and comparator), study population (age, sex, type of diabetes, visual acuity, type of DR, and other retinal diseases), HRQL instrument(s) used, and results for the outcomes of interest.

Assessment of Methodological Quality

Quality Assessment of HRQL Tools

For Key Question 1b, we used the COSMIN[29,36] checklist to assess the quality of the HRQL instruments. The checklist includes seven items: content and construct validity, internal consistency, reliability, absolute measurement error, responsiveness, and interpretability.[37] Each item is rated with the following options: "not done," or "low," "indeterminate," or "high" quality. Validity, reliability, and responsiveness depend on the setting and the population in which they are assessed. Therefore, descriptions of the study population characteristics, measurements, settings, and data analysis of every individual study were rated. If a description was lacking, the item was rated as indeterminate. One reviewer assessed the HRQL instruments in consultation with an expert in the HRQL field.

Quality Assessment for Included Studies

For Key Question 2, we assessed trials using the Cochrane Risk of Bias (ROB) tool for RCTs.[38] The ROB includes six domains which assess sequence generation, allocation concealment, blinding (participants and personnel, and outcome assessors), incomplete outcome data, selective outcome reporting, and other sources of bias. Each domain is assessed as "low," "unclear," or "high" based on the predefined criteria layed out the Cochrane Handbook, and the study is given an overall rating based on the assessment of each domain.

We used a modified version of the Newcastle-Ottawa Scale (NOS) for cohort studies.[39] The NOS includes seven items assessing sample selection, comparability of cohorts, and the assessment of outcomes. One star was allotted for each item that was adequately addressed in the study, with the exception of the comparability of cohorts, for which a maximum of two stars could be given. The overall score was calculated by tallying the stars, with a total possible score of eight stars.

The methodological quality of before-after studies was assessed using a modified version of the NOS that assessed sample selection and the assessment of outcomes. One star was allotted for each item that was adequately addressed in the study. The overall score was calculated by tallying the stars, with a total possible score of five stars.

Two reviewers (AM, CS, DD) independently assessed the methodological quality of the included studies. Decision rules were developed a priori through discussions with content and methodology experts. Discrepancies in quality assessment were resolved through consensus.

Data Analysis

For Key Question 1, we developed summary tables of the HRQL instruments, their characteristics, and their psychometric properties. For Key Question 2, we developed summary evidence tables of the study and population characteristics, and outcomes. Key Question 3 is presented in a descriptive analysis.

Mean differences (MD) and 95 percent confidence intervals (95% CI) were calculated for continuous variables. Missing means were approximated by medians. Missing standard deviations were computed from standard errors, confidence intervals, or p-values. If none of these were available, they were estimated from ranges or interquartile ranges, or imputed from other similar studies with the same outcome. We did not conduct any meta-analyses due to the heterogeneity of interventions and patient characteristics.

Grading the Evidence for Key Question 2

We used the EPC GRADE approach[40] to assess the strength of evidence for HRQL. The following four major domains were examined: risk of bias (incorporating both study design and study conduct), consistency, directness, and precision. An overall evidence grade based on the ratings for the individual domains was assigned. The overall strength of evidence was graded as "high" (indicating high confidence that the evidence reflects the true effect and further research is very unlikely to change our confidence in the estimate of effect); "moderate" (indicating moderate confidence that the evidence reflects the true effect and further research may change our confidence in the estimate of effect and may change the estimate); "low" (indicating low confidence that the evidence reflects the true effect and further research is likely to change our confidence in the estimate of effect and is likely to change the estimate); and "insufficient" (indicating that evidence is either unavailable or does not permit estimation of an effect). The strength of evidence was graded by one reviewer.

Results

Literature Review and Screening

The electronic literature search identified 6,961 unique citations. After the first level of screening based on title and abstract 6,441 articles were excluded from further review, leaving 520 articles for full-text retrieval. We identified an additional 14 studies through hand searching and contact with content experts. Of the 534 articles identified, 34 could not be located in either the University of Alberta libraries' holdings or through interlibrary loan requests. Of the 499 articles reviewed at the second level of screening, 16 addressed Key Question 1a. Eleven of these studies used validated measures to evaluate health-related quality of life (HRQL) and were applicable to Key Question 1b. Nine unique studies met our inclusion criteria to address Key Questions 2 and 3. Two of these studies[41,42] each had a related publication.[43,44] Figure 2 depicts the flow of the studies through the screening process and provides a breakdown of reasons for exclusion (see Appendix C for a list of excluded studies).

Figure 2. Flow diagram for study retrieval and selection

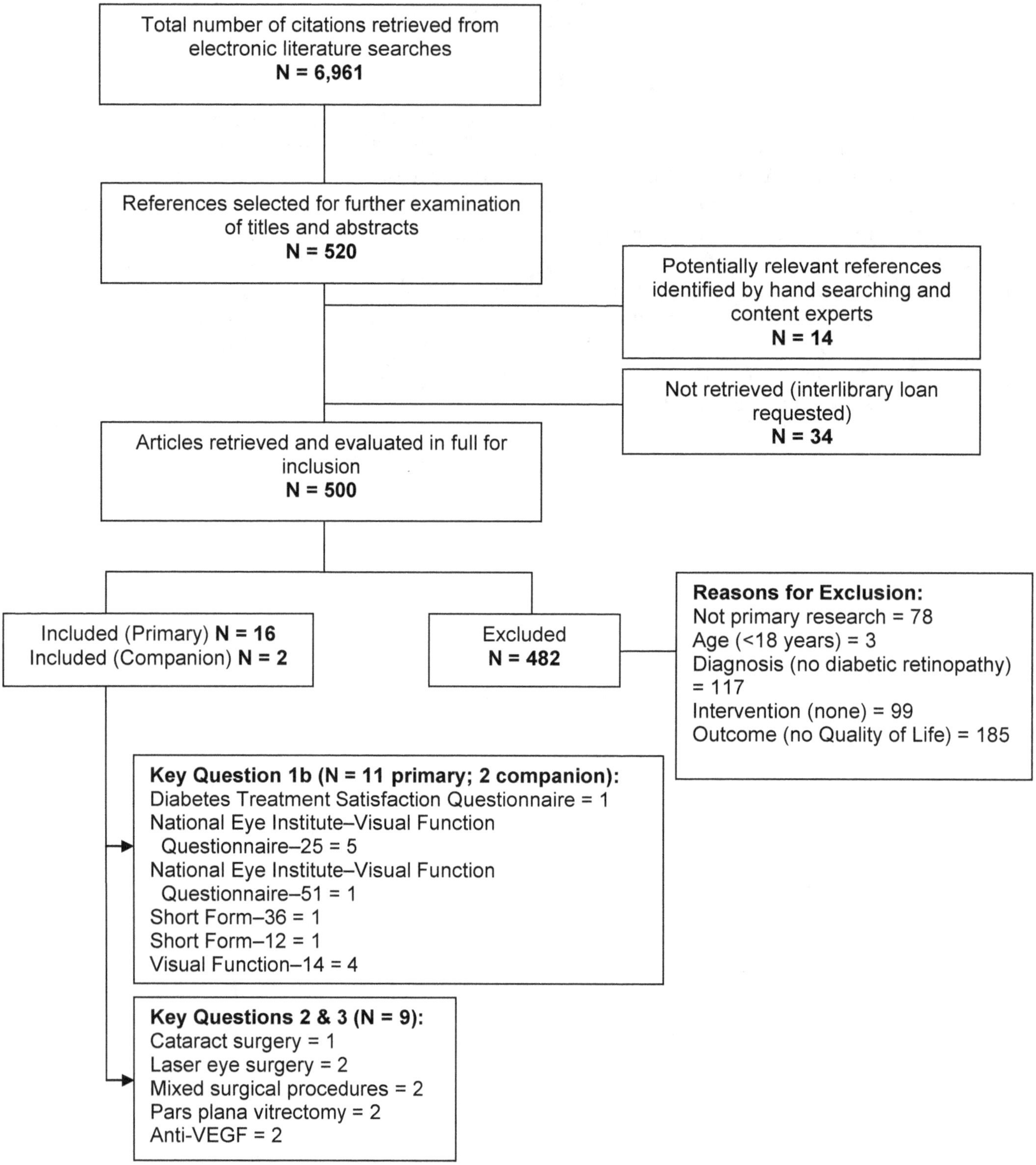

```
┌─────────────────────────────────────┐
│ Total number of citations retrieved │
│     from electronic literature      │
│              searches               │
│            N = 6,961                │
└─────────────────┬───────────────────┘
                  │
                  ▼
┌─────────────────────────────────────┐
│ References selected for further     │
│ examination of titles and abstracts │
│              N = 520                │
└─────────────────┬───────────────────┘
                  │
                  │        ┌──────────────────────────────────┐
                  ├────────│ Potentially relevant references  │
                  │        │ identified by hand searching and │
                  │        │         content experts          │
                  │        │              N = 14              │
                  │        └──────────────────────────────────┘
                  │
                  │        ┌──────────────────────────────────┐
                  ├────────│ Not retrieved (interlibrary loan │
                  │        │             requested)           │
                  │        │              N = 34              │
                  │        └──────────────────────────────────┘
                  ▼
┌─────────────────────────────────────┐
│ Articles retrieved and evaluated in │
│          full for inclusion         │
│              N = 500                │
└─────────────────┬───────────────────┘
```

- **Included (Primary) N = 16**
- **Included (Companion) N = 2**

- **Excluded N = 482**

Reasons for Exclusion:
Not primary research = 78
Age (<18 years) = 3
Diagnosis (no diabetic retinopathy) = 117
Intervention (none) = 99
Outcome (no Quality of Life) = 185

Key Question 1b (N = 11 primary; 2 companion):
Diabetes Treatment Satisfaction Questionnaire = 1
National Eye Institute–Visual Function
 Questionnaire–25 = 5
National Eye Institute–Visual Function
 Questionnaire–51 = 1
Short Form–36 = 1
Short Form–12 = 1
Visual Function–14 = 4

Key Questions 2 & 3 (N = 9):
Cataract surgery = 1
Laser eye surgery = 2
Mixed surgical procedures = 2
Pars plana vitrectomy = 2
Anti-VEGF = 2

Key Question 1a. What HRQL measures have been used in studies of treatments for diabetic retinopathy?

We identified four HRQL measures that have been used in studies assessing the treatment of diabetic retinopathy (DR). The most commonly used measure was the National Eye Institute Visual Functioning Questionnaire (VFQ), which is available in two versions. Five studies[41,42,45-47] used the 25 item version (VFQ–25); one[48] used the 51-item version (VFQ–51). In addition, seven recently completed trials that have not yet published their results reported using the VFQ–25 (See Appendix A for trial registration numbers). One study[49] used both the VFQ–25 and the Medical Outcomes Study (MOS) 36–Item Short Form Health Survey (SF–36). Two studies[50,51] used the Visual Function Index (VF–14). One study used both the VF–14 and the MOS 12-Item Short Form Health Survey (SF–12)[52], and another study[53] used the VF–14 plus a questionnaire to assess satisfaction with surgical outcomes. One study[54] used the Diabetes Treatment Satisfaction Questionnaire (DTSQ) plus a questionnaire to assess the degree to which treatment outcomes corresponded to patient expectations. One study[55] used qualitative interviews to assess quality of life but did not use a specific measure.

In addition to the measures used in studies of treatment for DR, we also identified two HRQL measures that have been developed specifically for patients with DR: the Retinopathy Treatment Satisfaction Questionnaire (RetTSQ), and the Retinopathy Dependent Quality of Life (RetDQoL) measure. Currently there is no literature describing their use in the evaluation of treatments for DR.

Key Question 1b. What are the psychometric properties of the HRQL measures used in the studies?

The six HRQL tools can be separated into two broad groups: generic tools and specific tools. The latter category can be further divided into tools developed for use in populations with: low vision, diabetes mellitus, and DR. See Appendix D for a description of the six measurement tools. Table 1 presents the psychometric properties of the measures. The ratings of the measurement properties based on the Consensus-based Standards for the selection of health Measurement INstruments (COSMIN) checklist are shown in Table 2. Below is a summary description of each tool.

Generic Assessment Tools

Medical Outcomes Study 36–Item Short Form Health Survey (SF–36)

The SF–36 is a 36 item questionnaire designed for use as a generic indicator of health status in clinical use, research, population surveys, and evaluative studies of health policy.[56] It incorporates physical, social, and mental concepts of both positive and negative aspects health. A higher score on the SF–36 represents better health. It has been used for evaluation in a variety of conditions and for comparisons of different populations including the general public.[57]

Reliability and validity of the SF–36 have been examined in both healthy and patient populations. Construct validity is good, and when compared with other health instruments (*Sickness Impact Profile, Quality of Well-being Scale, Nottingham Health Profile*), the SF–36 was more sensitive to change of community dwelling elderly persons, elderly patients, and patients with joint replacements.[58-60] However, the study by Matza[49] found that the SF–36 was unable to differentiate changes in visual acuity after treatment for DR, especially when compared with the VFQ–25.

Advantages of the SF–36 as compared to other generic instruments are its brevity and comprehensiveness. Limitations have been identified with validity pertaining to chronic disabilities, the severely ill, and the elderly. Some experts question the responsiveness of scores to changes in health status with certain populations, particularly: potential floor effects in the severely ill[56] and ceiling effects in healthy elderly people residing in the community.[60] Finally, the appropriateness of the SF–36 in the elderly is unclear[61] due to evidence that shows high percentages of missing data in this population.[59,62] Hayes and colleagues reported missing data in 70 percent of 122 respondents who were 75 years of age and older; however, they hypothesized this was likely related to visual or writing problems.[62]

Low-Vision Related Assessment Tools

National Eye Institute Visual Function Questionnaire-25-item version (VFQ–25)

The VFQ–25 is a reduced version of the National Eye Institute's 51-item VFQ developed to elicit patient perceptions of their visual impairment and its relation to HRQL. The VFQ–25 includes 1 general health item in addition to 11 visual subscale scores of: general vision, ocular pain, near vision, distance vision, social function, mental health, role limitations, dependency, driving, color vision, and peripheral vision. A high score on the VFQ–25 indicates better visual function and HRQL.[63] The reliability and validity of the VFQ–25 has been demonstrated in a variety of eye conditions including: cataracts, age-related macular degeneration, DR, primary open-angle glaucoma, and cytomegalovirus retinitis.[63] Furthermore, a strong association between the VFQ–25 and visual acuity has been demonstrated, independent of the degree of retinopathy.[64] A Japanese version of the VFQ–25 was used in the studies by Okamoto et al.,[41,43] and Emi et al.,[45,46] and has been shown to be reliable and valid in the Japanese population.[65]

Visual Function–14 (VF–14)

The VF–14 asks patients to assess their ability to perform 14 everyday activities that can be affected by cataracts. There are 18 items related to visual acuity including: reading, recognizing people, seeing steps, stairs or curbs, doing fine handwork, writing checks or filling out forms, playing games, taking part in sports, cooking, watching television, and driving. A higher score on the VF–14 indicates that the patient is better able to complete the everyday activities included in the questionnaire.[66] Boisjoly[50] found that in a variety of eye conditions, the VF–14 was more strongly correlated with changes in patients' self-reported visual trouble and satisfaction with vision than with changes in visual acuity and general outcome measures.

Diabetes-Related HRQL Assessment Tools

Diabetes Treatment Satisfaction Questionnaire (DTSQ)

The DTSQ measures patients' satisfaction with the treatment they receive for their diabetes. It has been designed for use only with persons with either type 1 or type 2 diabetes mellitus and has not been validated for use in the narrower population of patients with DR. Six items on the questionnaire are combined to provide a measure of treatment satisfaction; the remaining two items evaluate the perceived frequency of hyperglycemia and hypoglycemia. A high score on the DTSQ indicates the patient has a high level of satisfaction with their treatment.[67] The DTSQ can effectively measure psychological outcomes related to diabetes treatment and has demonstrated sensitivity to changes in patient satisfaction related to changes in diabetic interventions.[68]

Diabetic Retinopathy Related HRQL Assessment Tools

Diabetic Retinopathy Dependent Quality of Life (RetDQoL)

The RetDQoL is a recently developed tool designed to evaluate the QOL of patients diagnosed with DR and is modeled on the Audit of Diabetes-Dependent QoL.[69] The questionnaire begins with two broad questions related to present quality of life and what the patient's perceived QOL would be if they did not have diabetic eye problems. The remaining 24 items are specific questions related to aspects of QOL. Each item is split into two parts: part "a" asks the patient to evaluate the impact of the domain on their QOL; part "b" asks the patient to rank how important each domain is in their life. The RetDQoL has demonstrated high internal consistency and good construct validity.[70] The RetDQoL has not yet been used in clinical trials investigating the impact of an intervention for DR.

Diabetic Retinopathy Treatment Satisfaction Questionnaire (RetTSQ)

The RetTSQ is a recently developed tool designed to evaluate patients' satisfaction with the treatment they receive for their DR. The DTSQ was used as a model for the development of this questionnaire. The RetTSQ is comprised of 13 items relating to patient satisfaction with different areas of treatment for DR. The 13 items are split into two subscales: one used to evaluate positive aspects of treatment, and the other to evaluate negative aspects. A high score on the RetTSQ indicates a high level of satisfaction with treatment. The internal consistency of the RetTSQ has been demonstrated to be high, and construct validity to be good. The RetTSQ has not been used in any clinical trials to evaluate the impact of an intervention for DR.[71]

Table 1. Psychometric properties of health-related quality of life assessment tools used in studies of the treatment of diabetic retinopathy

Measure	Study population	Construct validity	Internal consistency	Test-retest reliability	Responsiveness
Generic HRQL assessment tools					
SF-36[56,57,72]	Patients who participated in the Medical Outcomes Study (1986) (US); differed in SES, medical and psychiatric dx and disease severity	7 scales (excluding general health) explain two-thirds of reliable variance in evaluations of current health status in UK, U.S., and Sweden; Scales have demonstrated 80–90% empirical validity in studies involving physical and mental health criteria compared with the longer MOS; Validity of each scale has been shown to differ from other scales: Physical functioning (r = 0.85), role-physical (r = 0.81) and bodily pain scales (r = 0.76) correlate most strongly with the PCS score, and are the most valid physical health measures; Mental health (r = 0.87), role-emotional (r = 0.78) and social functioning (r = 0.67) correlate most strongly with the MCS score and are the most valid mental measures	Median item-scale correlation (corrected for overlap) for each of the 8 scales ranged from 0.63 (general health) to 0.79 (mental health); all items except for general health (r = 0.38) exceeded the 0.40 standard for item-internal consistency; overall trends in item-internal consistency were replicated across patient subgroups; Median-item scale correlations for the 8 scales remained high across subgroups ranging from: 0.39 to 0.80	Each scale exceeded the minimum reliability standard of 0.70 for group comparisons; most reliability estimates for physical and mental summary scores exceed 0.80, and 0.90 for the PCS and MCS; Reliability ranged from 0.78 (general health) to 0.93 (physical functioning); Range for subgroups was 0.65 to 0.94	Mental health scale and MCS are useful in screening for psychiatric disorders (e.g. with a cut off score of 42, MCS has a sensitivity of 74% and a specificity of 81% to detect depressive disorder); 3 physical scales are the most responsive to benefits of knee and hip replacement, and heart valve surgery; 3 mental health scales are the most responsive in comparisons of pt before and after recovery from depression, change in severity of depression and treatment for depression

ADVS = Activities of Daily Vision Scale; BCVA = best corrected visual acuity; DR = diabetic retinopathy; dx = diagnosis; DTSQ = Diabetes Treatment Satisfaction Questionnaire; ETDRS = Early Treatment of Diabetic Retinopathy Study; HRQL = health-related quality of life; ICC = interclass correlation coefficient; MCS = mental component summary; mo = month; MOS = Medical Outcomes Study; PCS = physical component summary; pt = patient; QoL = quality of life; RetDQoL = Diabetic Retinopathy Dependent Quality of Life; RetTSQ = Diabetic Retinopathy Treatment Satisfaction Questionnaire; r/t = related to; SES = socioeconomic status; SIP = sickness impact profile; tx = treatment; US = United States; U.K. = United Kingdom; VA = Visual Acuity; VF = visual function; VFQ = National Eye Institute Visual Function Questionnaire

Table 1. Psychometric properties of health-related quality of life assessment tools used in studies of the treatment of diabetic retinopathy (continued)

Measure	Study population	Construct validity	Internal consistency	Test-retest reliability	Responsiveness
Low vision-related HRQL assessment tools					
VFQ–25[63,73]	VFQ–51—visually impaired persons with diverse eye conditions (N = 598 total; N with DR = 123; N pt included in test-retest reliability analysis = 96); VFQ–25—visual impaired persons with diverse eye conditions (N=859 [597 pt from previous study]; N with DR = 181)	VFQ–51—high correlations between VFQ scales and the VF–14 and ADVS: activity-oriented scales (near, distance vision and driving scale) and other vision-targeted scales: r = 0.9 to 0.6, p = 0.01; general vision ratings : r = 0.7, p < 0.001; mental distress ratings: r = 0.7, p = 0.001; significant correlation for peripheral and color vision with Visual Activities Questionnaire; poor correlation with most SF–36 scales, highest correlation between SF–36 mental component and VFQ–51 mental distress ratings: r = 0.4, p=0.001; correlations between VFQ-51 and ETDRS VA were moderate for scales that reflected the difficulty pt had with visual activities. VFQ–25—Correlations between the VFQ-25 subscales and VFQ-51 counterparts >0.90; correlations between responses on VFQ–25 and ETDRS visual acuity were in the range of 0.65 to 0.70 for subscales that reflected the degree of difficulty with visual activities related to general vision, near vision and distance vision; remaining subscales showed lower correlations ranging from 0.39 to 0.69 with the exception of the ocular pain subscale (lowest) between 0.06 to 0.11	VFQ–51—Cronbach's α for subscales range from 0.66 to 0.94; 86% of internal consistency estimates ≥ 0.7; VFQ–25—Subscale ranges from 0.71 to 0.85; among persons with eye disease, all 8 multi-item subscales had an internal consistency ≥0.70	VFQ–51—ICC for the 11 subscales range from 0.68 to 0.91	Scale scores improve with intervention; greater improvement in visual function is associated with greater improvement in HRQL; Correlations between responses on the VFQ-51 and ETDRS visual acuity were moderate for scales that reflect the degree of difficulty that a person has with common visual activities; Correlations between each of the scales and visual acuity in the better and worse eyes were similar in magnitude

ADVS = Activities of Daily Vision Scale; BCVA = best corrected visual acuity; DR = diabetic retinopathy; dx = diagnosis; DTSQ = Diabetes Treatment Satisfaction Questionnaire; ETDRS = Early Treatment of Diabetic Retinopathy Study; HRQL = health-related quality of life; ICC = interclass correlation coefficient; MCS = mental component summary; mo = month; MOS = Medical Outcomes Study; PCS = physical component summary; pt = patient; QoL = quality of life; RetDQoL = Diabetic Retinopathy Dependent Quality of Life; RetTSQ = Diabetic Retinopathy Treatment Satisfaction Questionnaire; r/t = related to; SES = socioeconomic status; SIP = sickness impact profile; tx = treatment; US = United States; U.K. = United Kingdom; VA = Visual Acuity; VF = visual function; VFQ = National Eye Institute Visual Function Questionnaire

Table 1. Psychometric properties of health-related quality of life assessment tools used in studies of the treatment of diabetic retinopathy (continued)

Measure	Study population	Construct validity	Internal consistency	Test-retest reliability	Responsiveness
VF–14[66,74]	Patients undergoing cataract surgery (N = 766); 522 pt of original population used to test responsiveness (had not received second surgery by 4 mo followup); 383 pt of original population used to test reproducibility (had not received second surgery by 12 mo followup)	Criterion validity assessed by examining the correlation between VF–14 scores and other measures of vision included visual acuity and global self-rating of the overall difficulty and satisfaction patients had with their vision; VF–14 with pt self-reported trouble with vision (r = -0.45) and overall satisfaction with vision (r = 0.34) higher than correlations with other vision measures; correlation between VF–14 score and visual acuity was strongest in the better eye (r = 0.27); VF–14 moderately correlated with SIP score (r = -0.39); and strongly correlated with VR-SIP score (r = -0.57)	Cronbach's α for total scale = 0.85; Cronbach's α for subscales ranged from 0.32 to 0.61	In pt whose 12 mo followup BCVA in each eye remained within 1 Snellen line of 4 mo followup value (n = 249) (mean VF–14 scores at 12 mo 1.5 points lower than 4 mo scores): ICC = 0.57; In pt with no difference between 12 mo and 4 mo followup BCVA (n = 96) (mean difference between 4 and 12 mo followup VF–14 scores = 1.7 points; p<0.05): ICC = 0.71; In pt with no complications (n = 47) (no significant difference in mean 4 and 12 mo followup scores): ICC = 0.76; Pt who had identical answers to 2 global questions r/t trouble and satisfaction with vision (n = 119) (mean VF–14 scores at 12 mo followup 1.1 points lower than 4 mo followup score; p<0.05): ICC = 0.79; After adjusting for pt who scored 100 points on VF–14 at both 4 and 12 mo: ICCs = 0.50 to 0.73	Pts who underwent cataract removal in one eye (up to 4 mo followup) (n = 522): effect size 1.02 for VF–14, -0.26 for SIP; Pt whose VA in operated eye improved by ≥ 2 Snellen lines: effect size 1.07 (VF–14), -0.29 (SIP)—results did not differ when patients stratified by baseline VA; Pt whose functional status improved at 4 mo followup (n = 510): effect size 1.06 (VF–14), -0.27 (SIP); Pt who reported an improved rating of amount of trouble with vision at 4 mo followup (n = 438): effect size: 1.17 (VF–14), -0.28 (SIP); Pt who reported improved rating of satisfaction with vision at 4 mo followup (n = 470): effect size: 1.14 (VF–14), -0.30 (SIP)

ADVS = Activities of Daily Vision Scale; BCVA = best corrected visual acuity; DR = diabetic retinopathy; dx = diagnosis; DTSQ = Diabetes Treatment Satisfaction Questionnaire; ETDRS = Early Treatment of Diabetic Retinopathy Study; HRQL = health-related quality of life; ICC = interclass correlation coefficient; MCS = mental component summary; mo = month; MOS = Medical Outcomes Study; PCS = physical component summary; pt = patient; QoL = quality of life; RetDQoL = Diabetic Retinopathy Dependent Quality of Life; RetTSQ = Diabetic Retinopathy Treatment Satisfaction Questionnaire; r/t = related to; SES = socioeconomic status; SIP = sickness impact profile; tx = treatment; US = United States; U.K. = United Kingdom; VA = Visual Acuity; VF = visual function; VFQ = National Eye Institute Visual Function Questionnaire

Table 1. Psychometric properties of health-related quality of life assessment tools used in studies of the treatment of diabetic retinopathy (continued)

Measure	Study population	Construct validity	Internal consistency	Test-retest Reliability	Responsiveness
Diabetes-related HRQL assessment tools					
DTSQ[75]	Pt with diabetes mellitus (n = 286); divided into 3 groups: CSII: continuous subcutaneous insulin infusion; ICT: intensified conventional therapy; CT: conventional therapy	Evidence of construct validity demonstrated in populations with diabetes mellitus (not DR) by relationships between treatment satisfaction and: being less overweight ($r = 0.19$; $p<0.05$); having better glycemic control ($r = -0.28$; $p<0.001$) and being optimistic about recent diabetes control ($r = 0.56$; $p<0.001$)	Cronbach's α for total scale = 0.76; When item: how many hypoglycemic experiences have you experienced recent was removed, α = 0.79 for total scale	No data	Low score indicates that level of satisfaction has increased during the year; if no change occurred, a score of 21 would be obtained; Significantly different scores on the 3 subscales obtained between CSII, ICT and CT: $F = 30.4$; df 2, 123; $p<0.001$; Significant interaction between CSII, ICT, and CT, and magnitude of subscale score: $F = 4.81$; df 4, 246; $p<0.001$)
Diabetic retinopathy-related HRQL assessment tools					
RetDQoL[70]	Patients with DR (N = 207)	Predefined hypotheses were tested: Greater visual impairment, advanced stages of DR, & additional impact of DME will lead to more negative impact on QoL: *confirmed*; Significant correlation with clinical variables for overview items I (present QoL) and II (retinopathy-specific QoL), and the AWI of domain-specific items: *confirmed with exception of stage of DR and item I*; Significant correlations between AWI and overview items I and II, with the strongest positive relationship between AWI and overview item II: *confirmed*; Small significant correlations with subscales of SF-12: *confirmed*; Small significant correlation with tx satisfaction as measured by RetTSQ: *confirmed*; No significant correlations with sociodemographic variables: *not confirmed for item I (living alone, employment, age, sex); confirmed for item II*	Cronbach's α weighted impact scores for all domains = 0.958; Cronbach's α for unweighted impact scores and the importance ratings = 0.96, 0.84, respectively	No data	No data

ADVS = Activities of Daily Vision Scale; BCVA = best corrected visual acuity; DME = diabetic macular edema; DR = diabetic retinopathy; dx = diagnosis; DTSQ = Diabetes Treatment Satisfaction Questionnaire; ETDRS = Early Treatment of Diabetic Retinopathy Study; HRQL = health-related quality of life; ICC = interclass correlation coefficient; MCS = mental component summary; mo = month; MOS = Medical Outcomes Study; PCS = physical component summary; pt = patient; QoL = quality of life; RetDQoL = Diabetic Retinopathy Dependent Quality of Life; RetTSQ= Diabetic Retinopathy Treatment Satisfaction Questionnaire; r/t = related to; SES = socioeconomic status; SIP = sickness impact profile; tx = treatment; US = United States; U.K. = United Kingdom; VA = Visual Acuity; VF = visual function; VFQ = National Eye Institute Visual Function Questionnaire

Table 1. Psychometric properties of health-related quality of life assessment tools used in studies of the treatment of diabetic retinopathy (continued)

Measure	Study population	Construct validity	Internal consistency	Test-retest Reliability	Responsiveness
RetTSQ[71]	Patients with DR (N = 207)	Predefined hypotheses were tested: Greater visual impairment, advanced stages of DR, & additional impact of DME are associated with less tx satisfaction: *confirmed*; Moderate significant correlations with subscales of SF–12: *confirmed*; Positive correlations between tx satisfaction and QOL scores on RetDQoL: *confirmed*; No significant correlations with sociodemographic variables: *confirmed*	Cronbach's α of total scale = 0.90; Cronbach's α for both of the subscales = 0.85	No data	No data

ADVS = Activities of Daily Vision Scale; BCVA = best corrected visual acuity; DR = diabetic retinopathy; dx = diagnosis; DTSQ = Diabetes Treatment Satisfaction Questionnaire; ETDRS = Early Treatment of Diabetic Retinopathy Study; HRQL = health-related quality of life; ICC = interclass correlation coefficient; MCS = mental component summary; mo = month; MOS = Medical Outcomes Study; PCS = physical component summary; pt = patient; QoL = quality of life; RetDQoL = Diabetic Retinopathy Dependent Quality of Life; RetTSQ = Diabetic Retinopathy Treatment Satisfaction Questionnaire; r/t = related to; SES = socioeconomic status; SIP = sickness impact profile; tx = treatment; US = United States; U.K. = United Kingdom; VA = Visual Acuity; VF = visual function; VFQ = National Eye Institute Visual Function Questionnaire

Table 2. Rating of the psychometric properties health-related quality of life assessment tools used in studies of treatment of diabetic retinopathy

Measure	Content validity	Construct validity	Internal consistency	Test re-test reliability	Measurement error	Responsiveness	Interpretability
SF–36	+	+	+	+	+	+	+
VFQ–25	+	+	+	+	0	?	?
VF–14	?	+	+	?	0	?	0
DTSQ	+	+	+	+	+	+	0
RetDQoL	+	+	+	0	0	0	0
RetTSQ	+	+	+	0	0	0	0

Method or result was rated as: += high quality; ?: indeterminate; -: low quality; 0: no data available

Key Questions 2 and 3: What is the evidence that HRQL is improved by any intervention; and what is the relationship between HRQL and any relevant variables?

Description of Included Studies

We identified two RCTs and seven observational studies that addressed Key Questions 2 and 3. The population and study characteristics are summarized in Table 3. Additional population and study characteristics are available in Appendix F.

The two RCTs[42,47] were multicenter trials that recruited patients in Australia, North and South America, Europe, India, and Turkey. The trials examined two anti-VEGF treatments in patients with DME. The RESTORE study[47] was a three-arm double-masked RCT (n = 345) that compared ranibizumab monotherapy versus ranibizumab plus laser versus laser. The Macugen 1013 study[42] (n = 260) was a double-masked RCT comparing pegaptanib sodium versus sham.

For the observational studies, the interventions included laser photocoagulation,[48,54] vitrectomy,[41,45,46] panretinal photocoagulation,[46] and phacoemulsification cataract surgery for diabetic patients with cataracts.[51,53] Sample sizes ranged from 55 to 345 (IQR: 77 – 293.5). As a post hoc analysis, we examined the subgroup of patients with DME. Six studies[41,42,45,47,48,54] reported some results for those with DME. Two studies[51,53] included patients with DME, but did not report separate results. Patients with DME represented less than five percent of the study sample in these studies. One study[46] did not report whether patients with DME were included in their study.

Methodological Quality

Both RCTs were assessed as "unclear" risk of bias. The primary concern for both trials was incomplete outcome data and the use of the last observation carried forward approach for missing data. For the Macugen 1013 study,[42] all other domains were assessed as low risk of bias. For the RESTORE study,[47] the domains for allocation concealment, blinding of HRQL assessment, and baseline balance for HRQL were assessed as unclear; the remaining domains were low risk of bias. Both trials received industry funding.

There were four cohort studies[41,46,51,53] and three before-after studies.[45,48,54] All data were collected prospectively. The methodological quality of the cohort studies was assessed as good for one[51] (7/8 stars), moderate for one[53] (6/8 stars), and low for two (3 or 4 of 8 stars). Two studies[53,54] enrolled patients that were rated to be truly or somewhat representative of average patients in the community, and the nonexposed cohort was drawn from the same community. For the remaining two studies, there was no description of the derivation of the cohort. All studies ascertained the exposure status from a secure source, most commonly from patient records. Two studies[53,54] controlled for potential confounders through multivariate analyses. All studies used a validated tool for outcome assessment. Two studies[46,51] had a followup duration of at least 6 months. For all studies, the rate of followup was either complete or considered unlikely to introduce bias.

The methodological quality of the before-after studies was assessed as good for one[54] (5/5 stars) and moderate for two[45,48] (4/5 stars). Two studies[45,54] enrolled patients that were rated to be truly or somewhat representative of average patients in the community. All studies ascertained the exposure status from a secure source, most commonly from patient records. All used a validated tool for outcome assessment. Two studies[45,54] had a followup duration of at least 6 months. For all three studies, the rate of followup was either complete or unlikely to introduce bias.

Overall this collection of observational studies is at high risk of bias due to weak study designs (before-after and cohort studies).

Results

The results are grouped by the type of intervention (e.g., anti-VEGF, laser photocoagulation). Three observational studies[41,48,54] conducted multivariate analyses to identify variables associated with HRQL outcomes; these results are presented with their respective studies. Table 4 summarizes the outcomes.

Anti-VEGF

From September 2005 to November 2009, the Macugen 1013 Study group[42] conducted a multicenter trial that investigated the efficacy of pegaptanib sodium versus sham injections. All patients were diagnosed with DME. Patients were randomized to receive 0.3 mg of pegaptanib sodium (n=133) or a sham treatment designed to mimic the intravitreal injection process (n=127). The primary efficacy endpoint was the number of patients who gained 10 letters or more on visual acuity compared to baseline. At 54 weeks after baseline 49 of 133 (36.8 percent) patients treated with pegaptanib had achieved an improvement of 10 or more letters, compared with 25 of 127 (19.7 percent) in the sham injection group. The odds ratio was 2.38 (95% CI, 1.32 to 4.30, p=0.0047). Additionally, patients who received pegaptanib reported statistically (p<0.05) and clinically significant (>5 point difference) improvements on the VFQ–25 at 54 weeks on the near vision, distant vision, and social functioning subscales. The change in composite score was not statistically significant. At 102 weeks after baseline, patients who received pegaptanib reported statistically (p<0.05) and clinically significant (>5 point difference) improvements on the composite score, and the distance vision, social functioning and mental health subscores compared with patients treated with a sham injection.

The RESTORE Study group[47] conducted a multicenter trial that investigated the efficacy of ranibizumab with and without laser treatment. All patients were diagnosed with DME. Patients were randomized to recieve 0.5 mg of ranibizumab plus sham laser treatment (n=116), 0.5 mg of ranibizumab plus laser treatment (n=118), and sham treatment plus laser treatment (n=111). The mean change in best corrected visual acuity (BCVA) from baseline to 12 months was the primary outcome. For patients treated with ranibizumab alone, 22.6 percent achieved a BCVA letter score of 15 or more, and 53 percent attained a BCVA letter score level more than 73 (20/40 Snellen equivalent); whereas 22.9 percent and 44.9 percent, respectively achieved those gains among the patients treated with ranibizumab plus laser therapy. Of patients who received laser treatment, 8.2 percent improved 15 or more letters on BCVA, and 23.6 percent reached a BVCA letter score more than 73. Scores on the VFQ–25 were significantly improved from baseline to 12 months for patients treated with ranibizumab alone and patients treated with ranibizumab in combination with laser compared with patients with laser treatment only. For the ranibizumab monotherapy group the composite score increased by 5.0 points compared with an increase of 0.6 for the laser treatment group (p=0.014). Similarly for the ranibizumab plus laser treatment group, the composite score increased by 5.4 points (p=0.004). Furthermore, at 12 months ratings of good to excellent vision were reported by 46 percent of patients treated with ranibizumab alone and 50 percent of those treated with ranibizumab plus laser treatment. This compares with

22 percent of patients who received only laser treatment. The proportion of patients reporting excellent to good vision at baseline were similar across the three groups—21 percent (ranibizumab), 23 percent (ranibizumab plus laser treatment), and 24 percent (laser only).

Laser photocoagulation

Tranos et al.[48] conducted a prospective study that followed 55 patients with DME. Best corrected visual acuity for distance vision and near vision were recorded as the number of letters read correctly on Early Treatment of Diabetic Retinopathy Study (ETDRS) charts at 4 meters and 40 centimeters, respectively. The mean baseline visual acuity was 42.7±8.4 (distance) and 56.4±9.1 (near). Patients completed the VFQ–51 prior to and 3 months following the last session of laser treatment. At the end of the followup period, DME had resolved in 46 (84 percent) patients, although improvement in visual acuity was small. Based on the VFQ–51, laser treatment resulted in an improvement in patients' perceived functional status and QOL. The composite score and the subscale scores associated with general vision, near vision, distance vision, vision-specific mental health, expectations for visual function, and dependency due to vision were significantly improved following laser treatment.

Multivariate models showed that improvement of the VFQ–51 composite score was associated with age less than 65 years ($p = 0.04$), number of laser spots (indicating more extensive treatment; $p = 0.02$), and worse vision-related QOL prior to laser treatment ($p = 0.03$). There was no statistically significant association between change in the composite score and stage of DR or duration of diabetes.

From June 2002 to March 2004, Mozaffarieh et al.[54] followed 105 patients undergoing first photocoagulation treatment for DME (n = 49) or proliferative diabetic retinopathy (PDR) (n = 56). Patients had laser treatments at 4 and 9 months, and then a final examination 12 months after the initial laser treatment. Best-corrected visual acuity was recorded using a Snellen chart, and visual acuity improvement was defined as the difference between the pre- and post-treatment logarithm of minimal angle of resolution (logMAR) acuity. All patients completed the DTSQ after their initial and final (9 month) laser treatments. Nine months after initial photocoagulation treatment 24.7 percent of all patients reported improvement in visual acuity. Vision remained the same in 71.4 percent and worse in 3.8 percent. These values remained constant 12 months after initial treatment for all but one patient whose vision deteriorated further. There was no statistically significant difference in vision improvement between patients with DME and PDR. Based on a maximum possible score of 36, satisfaction after the final (9 month) laser treatment was high (mean score = 27.9±5.2), with 42.8 percent scoring 31 or higher. Results of the DTSQ were not reported separately for the two groups of patients.

The Spearman correlation between treatment satisfaction and the patients' visual acuity after laser treatment for patients with DME and PDR was modest ($r = 0.28$–0.33, $p>0.2$). Satisfaction was associated with age, with older patients being more satisfied than younger patients (Spearman coefficient $r = 0.41$–0.56, $p<0.001$).

Vitrectomy

In a prospective study, Okamoto et al.[41] investigated vision-related QOL in 299 patients undergoing pars plana vitrectomy for various vitreoretinal disorders. The authors reported results separately for patients with PDR (n = 99) and DME (n = 38). The logMAR best corrected visual acuity and letter contrast sensitivity were obtained preoperatively and at 3 months postoperatively. All patients completed the VFQ–25 (Japanese version) before and 3 months after surgery. One hundred healthy volunteers who served as normal control subjects also completed the VFQ–25. Vitrectomy significantly improved visual acuity and contrast sensitivity in both patient groups. For patients with PDR, the composite VFQ–25 score and most subscale scores improved significantly following vitrectomy. The composite score gained 10.8±18.3 points. For those with DME, the change in the composite score was 6.0±20.8, but was not statistically significant. The only vision related subscales that showed statistically significant improvements for patients with DME were general vision, near activities, mental health, and peripheral vision. The composite score for the normal controls was 85.0±9.1, which is statistically significantly higher than the preoperative and postoperative composite scores in patients with PDR and DME.

Multiple regression analysis showed that improvement in contrast sensitivity was significantly correlated with changes in the VFQ–25 composite score for patients with PDR and DME. There was no significant correlation between changes in the VFQ–25 and postoperative visual acuity.

Emi et al.[45] followed 87 patients with DR. Of these, 41 (47 percent) had vitreous hemorrhage, 28 (32 percent) had DME, and 18 (21 percent) had fibrovascular membrane. All patients completed the VFQ–25 (Japanese version) 1 month before and 6 months after vitrectomy. At 6 months, 35 (85 percent) patients with vitreous hemorrhage reported that their visual acuity had improved; the remaining patients reported visual acuity as unchanged (n = 4) or worse (n = 2). For patients with DME and fibrovascular membrane, 9 (32 percent) and 13 (72 percent) reported improved visual acuity, respectively. For all patients, the mean VFQ–25 following vitrectomy increased in all 12 subscales; however, the changes were not statistically significant. Only the subgroup of patients with vitreous hemorrhage reported statistically significant improvements for 10 of the 12 subscales of the VFQ–25. For the subgroup of patients with fibrovascular membrane, the only subscale that had a statistically significant change from baseline was general vision.

Vitrectomy and panretinal photocoagulation

In a second study by Emi et al.,[46] 327 patients with DR were followed for 1 year. Of these, 136 (42 percent) underwent vitrectomy, 60 (18 percent) received panretinal photocoagulation, and 131 (40 percent) did not have any treatment and served as a comparison group. All patients completed the VFQ–25 (Japanese version) at the time of entry into the study and 1 year later. Visual acuity was reported as the logMAR score for the right and the left eyes. For the vitrectomy group, the VFQ–25 composite score improved by eight points and the change was statistically significant. Changes in the composite scores for the comparison group and the photocoagulation group were not statistically significant. At baseline, the VFQ–25 composite score for the vitrectomy group was significantly lower than that of either of the other groups; at 1 year followup, there was no statistically significant difference between the vitrectomy and the photocoagulation groups.

Phacoemulsification

From May 2001 to May 2003, Mozaffarieh et al.[53] prospectively evaluated visual outcomes and visual function after first-eye phacoemulsification cataract surgery. A total of 67 patients with different stages of DR were included: 17 patients had no apparent DR (group 1), 19 had mild nonproliferative diabetic retinopathy (NPDR) (group 2), 16 had moderate/severe NPDR (group 3), and 15 had proliferative diabetic retinopathy (PDR) (group 4). Patients were followed for 3 months after surgery. All patients completed the VF–14 prior to and 3 months after surgery. Three months postoperatively, 94.2 percent of patients reported improved visual acuity and 92.5 percent reported improvements in visual function. Improvements in both visual acuity and visual function decreased as the baseline level of retinopathy increased. Patients with no DR or mild retinopathy (groups 1 and 2) demonstrated significantly greater improvements in visual acuity and visual function compared with patients with more advanced DR (group 3 and 4).

From May 2000 to March 2004, Mozaffarieh et al.[51] followed 89 diabetic patients with bilateral cataracts. Of these, 66 had DR (mild NPDR: 35 percent, moderate/severe NPDR: 33 percent, PDR: 32 percent). Forty-one patients had surgery on one eye (group 1), and 48 had subsequent surgery on the second eye (group 2) at least 6 months later. Patients completed the VF–14 prior to surgery and 1, 3, 6, 8, and 12 months postoperatively. Patients with PDR had the lowest VF–14 scores at baseline and improved marginally over the study period regardless of whether they had surgery on one or both eyes (improvement of 2.6±10.8 points and 2.4±5.2 at 6 months, and 4.6±7.3 and -2.98±7.4 (decrease) at 12 months, respectively). A similar pattern was seen for patients with moderate/severe NPDR with an increase of 7.8±8.0 points and 6.2±5.6 at 6 months and 5.2±8.2 and -6.85±15.3 (decrease) at 12 months, respectively. For patients with no or mild NPDR, maximum VF–14 scores at 12 months followup were significantly higher than patients with more severe DR.

The impact of first-eye cataract surgery on QOL was evident in patients with no or mild DR with the highest VF–14 scores being achieved by 91.3 percent of patients in the first month. In contrast, for those with more severe DR 79.1 percent achieved the highest VF–14 score after 3 months.

In patients with no or mild DR who underwent second-eye surgery the improved functional status achieved after first surgery was sustained. For those who did not have second-eye surgery VF–14 scores decreased after 8 and 12 months. For those with more advanced levels of DR, there were no significant gains after second eye surgery at 12 months.

Table 3. Study characteristics and outcomes for studies reporting the impact of interventions for diabetic retinopathy on HRQL

Author Year Study design Country	Intervention HRQL measure Followup	Participants	Visual acuity outcomes	HRQL outcomes
Anti-VEGF				
Mitchell 2011[47] RCT Multicenter (73 centers in Australia, Canada, Europe, Turkey)	G1—ranibizumab 0.5 mg + sham laser G2—ranibizumab 0.5 mg + laser G3—laser + sham injection VFQ-25 3 mo, 12 mo	G1 = 116 G2 = 118 G3 = 111 DME = 345 (100%)	Median change in BCVA from baseline to 12 mo: G1 = 6.1±6.43 G2 = 5.9±7.92 G3 = 0.8±8.59 Median change in BCVA from baseline to 12 mo: G1 = 6.1 (-10.9–25.2) G2 = 6.0 (-26.7–27.6) G3 = 1.3 (-37.8–26.8) 95% CI for the mean change: G1 = 4.9, 7.3 G2 = 4.4, 7.3 G3 = -0.8, 2.4	VFQ-25, composite score at 12 mo G1—baseline: NR; improvement: 5.0 (p=0.014 compared to G3) G2—baseline: NR; improvement: 5.4 (p=0.004 compared to G3) G3—baseline: NR; improvement: 0.6 (NR) Other domains: G1—significant improvement for general vision, near vision activities, distance activities; other domains: NR G2— significant improvement for general vision, near vision activities, distance activities; other domains: NR G3—baseline: NR; no significant change from baseline
Sultan 2011[42] RCT Multicenter (60 centers in Australia, Europe, India, North America, South America)	G1—pegaptanib 0.3 mg G2—sham injection VFQ-25 baseline, 18, 54 & 102 wk	G1 = 133 G2 = 127 DME = 260 (100%)	% improvement of ≥10 letters from baseline at 54 wk: G1 = 43/133 (36.8%) G2 = 25/127 (19.7%) Odds ratio (95% CI) = 2.38 (1.32, 4.30); p=0.0047 % improvement of ≥10 letters from baseline at 102 wk G1 = 41/107 (38.3%) G2 = 30/100 (30%) Odds ratio (95% CI) = 1.57 (0.83, 2.97); p=0.1729	VFQ-25, composite score at 54 wk: G1—70.4; improvement 4.5 G2—69.2; improvement 1.3 Between group differences—2.92; range - 0.32 to 6.16 (p = 0.077) VFQ-25, composite score at 102 wk (n = 207): G1—69.8; improvement 4.6 G2—66.2; improvement 0.1 Between group differences—4.47; range - 0.26 to 8.68 (p = 0.038) Other domains: 54 wk: G1 vs. G2 had significantly more improvement for near vision activities, distance activities, social functioning; no difference for other domains 102 wk: G1 vs. G2 had significantly more improvement for distance activities, social functioning, mental health; no difference for other domains

95% CI = 95 percent confidence interval; BCVA = best corrected visual acuity; DR = diabetic retinopathy; DTSQ = Diabetes Treatment Satisfaction Questionnaire; DME = diabetic macular edema; mg = milligram; mo = month; NPDR = nonproliferative diabetic retinopathy; PDR = proliferative diabetic retinopathy; VF-14 = Visual Function-14; VFQ = National Eye Institute Visual Function Questionnaire; wk = week; yr = year

Table 3. Study characteristics and outcomes for studies reporting the impact of interventions for diabetic retinopathy on HRQL (continued)

Author Year Study design Country	Intervention HRQL measure Followup	Participants	Visual acuity outcomes	HRQL outcomes
Laser photocoagulation				
Tranos 2004[48] Before-after United Kingdom	Laser photocoagulation VFQ-51 3 mo	DME = 55 (100%) Mild NPDR = 13 Moderate NPDR = 32 Severe NPDR = 10	Binocular vision—baseline: 48.7±6.7 Distance vision—baseline: 42.7±8.4 letters; improvement: 2.2±6.2 Near vision—baseline: 56.4±9.1 letters; improvement: 2.1±5.0	Composite score—baseline: 77.9±17.6; improvement: 4.9±8.9 (p<0.001); Subscales—statistically significant improvement on 8 of 11 vision-related domains
Mozaffarieh 2005b Before-after Austria	Laser photocoagulation DTSQ 9 mo	Total = 105 PDR = 56 (53%) DME = 49 (47%)	24.7% reported improvement in visual acuity; 71.4% were unchanged; 3.8% were worse No difference in improvement between patients with PDR or DME	Mean± SD = 27.9±5.2 (maximum possible score = 36)
Vitrectomy				
Emi 2008[45] Before-after Japan	Vitrectomy VFQ-25 (Japanese version) 6 mo	DR = 87 (total) G1—vitreous hemorrhage = 41 G2—DME = 28 G3—fibrovascular membrane = 18	G1—improved: 35; unchanged: 4; worse: 2 G2—improved: 9; unchanged: 16; worse: 3 G3—improved: 13; unchanged: 3; worse: 2	G1—statistically significant improvement on 10 of 12 subscales G2—no statistically significant change from baseline on any subscales G3—only the general vision subscale had a statistically significant improvement from baseline
Okamoto 2010[41] Prospective cohort Japan	Pars plana vitrectomy VFQ-25 (Japanese version) 3 mo	G1—PDR = 99 G2—DME = 38 G3—normal controls = 100 Note: this is part of a larger study (n = 399) of patients with vitreoretinal disorders—retinal vein occlusion (32), macular hole (42), epiretinal membrane (33), retinal detachment (55)	logMAR G1—baseline: 1.37±0.75; 3 mo: 0.53±0.62 (p < 0.0001) G2—baseline = 0.76±0.49; 3 mo: 0.55±0.51 (p < 0.01) Contrast sensitivity G1—baseline: 5.4±7.2; 3 mo: 14.0±7.9 (p < 0.0001) G2—baseline 9.2±6.5; 3 mo: 12.7±7.1 (p < 0.0001)	G1—baseline: 52.8±19.0; 3 mo: 63.6±17.5 (p <0.001); Subscales—statistically significant improvement on 9/11 vision-related domains G2—baseline: 53.0±20.5; 3 mo: 59.0±21.0 (p = 0.84); Subscales—statistically significant improvement on 4/11 vision-related domains G3—85.0±9.1

Table 3. Study characteristics and outcomes for studies reporting the impact of interventions for diabetic retinopathy on HRQL (continued)

Author Year Study design Country	Intervention HRQL measure Followup	Participants	Visual acuity outcomes	HRQL outcomes
Vitrectomy and panretinal photocoagulation				
Emi 2009[46] Prospective cohort Japan	G1—vitrectomy G2—panretinal photocoagulation G3—no treatment VFQ-25 (Japanese version) 1 yr	G1 = 136 G2 = 60 G3 = 131	*logMAR—right eye* G1—baseline: 0.21; 1 yr: 0.46 (p < 0.001) G2—baseline: 0.64; 1 yr: 0.52 (p = 0.272) G3—baseline: 1.09; 1 yr: 1.06 (p = 0.294) *logMAR—left eye* G1—baseline: 0.19; 1 yr: 0.38 (p < 0.001) G2—baseline: 0.61; 1 yr: 0.56 (p = 0.081) G3—baseline: 1.10; 1 yr: 1.09 (p = 0.704)	*Composite score* G1—baseline: 67.4±17.3; 1 yr: 75.4±17.5 (p<0.001) G2—baseline: 80.7±15.7; 1 yr: 77.6±19.1 (p=0.113) G3—baseline: 91.3±7.8; 1 yr: 92.2±7.8 (p=0.169)
Phacoemulsification cataract surgery				
Mozaffarieh 2005a[53] Prospective cohort Austria	Phacoemulsification cataract surgery VF-14 3 mo	Cataracts = 67 (total) G1—no DR = 17 G2—mild NPDR = 19 G3—moderate/severe NPDR = 16 G4—PDR = 15	*logMAR (range)* G1—baseline: 0.62 (0.30–1.30); improvement 0.55 (0.30–1.15) G2—baseline: 0.60 (0.30–1.30); improvement 0.50 (0.30–1.08) G3—baseline: 0.67 (0.30–1.30); improvement 0.26 (0.15–0.48) G4—baseline: 0.71 (0.40–1.30); improvement 0.15 (-0.70–0.60)	G1—baseline: 52.21 (32.14–78.57); improvement 42.33 (21.43–60.71) G2—baseline: 55.92 (30.36–85.71); improvement 36.00 (12.50–58.93) G3—baseline: 46.65 (30.36–64.29); improvement 9.26 (1.79–25.00) G4—baseline: 40.12 (25.00–67.86); improvement 5.00 (-25.00–25.00)
Mozaffarieh 2009[51] Prospective cohort Austria	Phacoemulsification cataract surgery G1—first-eye surgery G2—both eyes VF-14 12 mo	Cataracts = 89 (total) No DR = 23 Mild NPDR = 23 Moderate NPDR = 22 PDR = 21	G1 & G2—patients with no or mild NPDR had greater improvement in visual acuity	G1 baseline: no DR: 59.3±12.4; mild 39.3±5.2; severe 40.9±8.6; PDR 35.3±4.4 6 mo: no DR: 96.8±2.0; mild 86.5±13.6; severe 48.8±6.7; PDR 37.9±14.0 12 mo: no DR: 79.5±5.5; mild 72.2±8.3; severe 46.1±10.7; PDR 39.9±9.0 G2 baseline: no DR 46.8±8.7; mild 63.4±16.3; severe 54.6±8.8; PDR 50.6±11.4 6 mo: no DR: 93.0±4.3; mild 94.6±2.5; severe 60.9±6.6; PDR 53.0±10.9 12 mo: no DR: 95.3±1.9; mild 95.3±2.2; severe 47.8±16.0; PDR 47.6±15.0

Summary of Findings

Anti-VEGF. Two RCTs provided data. In one RCT, 133 patients received 0.3 mg of pegaptanib sodium versus 127 patients who received a sham injection. All patients were diagnosed with DME. At 54 weeks there was no statistically significant difference between groups in the composite score on the VFQ–25. At 102 weeks, patients receiving pegaptanib sodium reported statistically significant improvements in the composite score. The second RCT was a three-arm trial comparing 0.5 mg of ranibizumab plus sham laser treatment (n=116), 0.5 mg of ranibizumab plus laser treatment (n=118), and sham treatment plus laser treatment (n=111). All patients were diagnosed with DME. The composite score on the VFQ–25 was significantly improved for patients treated with ranibizumab alone, or in combination with laser treatment compared with patients with laser treatment only. The strength of evidence for anti-VEGF is low. Further research is likely to change the confidence in the estimate of effect and is likely to change the estimate.

Laser photocoagulation. Two before-after studies provided data. In one study, 105 patients with PDR and DME reported high scores on the DTSQ at 9 months following surgery. In the second study, 110 patients with DME and NPDR reported a statistically significant improvement in HRQL at 3 months following surgery. While HRQL improved following surgery, the strength of evidence is insufficient to draw conclusions about the effect of laser photocoagulation in improving HRQL.

Vitrectomy. One cohort study and one before-after study provided data. In the cohort study, 99 patients with PDR reported a statistically significant improvement on the VFQ–25 (Japanese version) at 3 months following surgery. For those with DME (n = 38), the score improved, but the change was not statistically significant. The score on the VFQ–25 for the normal control group was significantly higher than the preoperative and postoperative scores of patients with PDR and DME. In the before-after study, 41 patients with vitreous hemorrhage reported statistically significant improvements on the VFQ–25 (Japanese version) at 6 months following surgery. This contrasts with patients with DME (n = 28) and fibrovascular membrane (n = 18) who reported no significant change in HRQL. While HRQL improved for some subgroups of patients, the strength of evidence is insufficient to draw conclusions about the effect of vitrectomy in improving HRQL.

Vitrectomy and panretinal photocoagulation. One cohort study provided data for 327 patients with DR. Of these, 136 underwent vitrectomy, 60 received panretinal photocoagulation, and 131 had no treatment and served as a comparison group. For the vitrectomy group, there was a statistically significant improvement in the VFQ–25 (Japanese version) composite score at 1 year following surgery. Changes in the VFQ–25 scores for the comparison group and the photocoagulation group were not statistically significant. The strength of evidence is insufficient to draw conclusions about the relative effect of vitrectomy versus panretinal photocoagulation in improving HRQL.

Phacoemulsification for cataract surgery. Two cohort studies provided data. One study evaluated visual function using the VF–14 after first-eye phacoemulsification cataract surgery. Three months following surgery, 94 percent of patients reported improved visual acuity and 93 percent reported improvements in visual function. Patients with no or mild DR demonstrated significantly greater improvements in visual acuity and function compared with patients with more advanced disease. The second study followed 89 diabetic patients with bilateral cataracts. At 12 months following surgery, patients with PDR had the lowest VF–14 scores at baseline and improved marginally over the study period regardless of whether they had cataract surgery on one or both eyes. A similar pattern was seen for patients with moderate/severe NPDR. For patients with no or mild NPDR, maximum VF–14 scores at 12 months were significantly higher than for patients with more severe DR. While HRQL improved, the strength of evidence is insufficient to draw conclusions about the effect of this surgery in improving HRQL.

Factors associated with outcomes. No conclusions can be drawn about factors associated with HRQL outcomes. In one study, multivariate analysis found that age <65 years, more severe level of DR, and low preoperative QOL were associated with improved HRQL following laser photocoagulation. In another study that also investigated laser photocoagulation, univariate analysis showed an association between age and treatment satisfaction, with older patients (>65 years) being more satisfied. In a study of vitrectomy, multivariate analysis showed that improvement in contrast sensitivity was significantly correlated with changes in the VFQ–25 for patients with PDR and DME. There was no significant correlation between VFQ–25 and visual acuity.

Table 4. Strength of evidence for health-related quality of life outcomes

Design # studies (sample size)	Risk of Bias	Consistency	Directness	Precision	Strength of evidence
Anti-VEGF					
2 RCTs (n = 605)	Medium	Inconsistent (at 1 yr)	Direct	Not pooled	Low
Laser photocoagulation					
2 before-after studies (n = 160)	High	Unknown (single study)	Direct	Not pooled	Insufficient
Vitrectomy					
1 cohort study (n = 237) 1 before-after study (n = 87)	High	Consistent	Direct	Not pooled	Insufficient
Vitrectomy and panretinal photocoagulation					
1 cohort study (n = 327)	High	Unknown (single study)	Direct	Not pooled	Insufficient
Phacoemulsification cataract surgery					
2 cohort studies (n = 156)	Medium	Consistent	Direct	Not pooled	Insufficient

Discussion

Using a comprehensive search strategy and concerted efforts to avoid publication and selection bias, this review identified the evidence on the effect that interventions for DR or DME have on HRQL. Overall we identified four measures—one generic, two vision-specific, and one diabetes-specific—that have been used to measure HRQL in studies of treatment for DR. As well, we identified two recently developed tools that are specific to patients with DR. We identified two RCTs and seven observational studies involving between 55 and 345 patients that addressed the question of whether HRQL is improved for any intervention for DR or DME.

HRQL Measures

Only one generic HRQL measure has been used to assess the impact that interventions for DR have on HRQL in patients with DR. The SF–36 gathers information about the patient's perceived health and asks about eight health concepts: physical functioning (ability to perform physical activities), physical role functioning (problems with daily tasks due to physical health), bodily pain (degree of limitation due to pain), general health (personal perception of health), vitality (degree of energy—tired and worn out to full of energy), social function (ability to perform social activities), emotional role functioning (problems with daily tasks due to mental health), and mental health (overall emotional state).[50] Generic HRQL tools are generally insensitive to the presence of specific eye disease. Furthermore, the SF–36 appears to be unresponsive to changes in visual acuity in patients with DR.[49] The authors suggest that this may be because the SF–36 assesses a wide range of characteristics that are not directly related to visual acuity. Other generic measures that include assessment of vision function (e.g., the Health Utilities Index[76]) may be a reasonable choice for researchers to consider if a generic health status measure is needed. Generic HRQL tools can be used to make comparisons with the general population (regardless of the underlying condition), estimate the relative impact of various medical conditions, and derive a utility value summarizing health status for cost-effectiveness modeling.[20,23,49] The decision to use a generic measure along with a specific measure needs to be driven by the purpose of the measurement.[35]

Two validated and clinically responsive vision-specific measures, the VFQ–25 and VF–14, have been used to measure the impact of different interventions on HRQL in individuals with DR. Vision-specific measures have been shown to be sensitive to differences in vision status and functioning among patients with DR.[50,63,64,66]

The diabetes-specific tool, the DTSQ, was specifically developed to measure satisfaction with treatment regimens in individuals with diabetes. Research has shown that satisfaction with treatment is associated with compliance with treatment.[77,78] The DTSQ was not designed to measure satisfaction with other aspects of the diabetes care and management.[67] It is most useful when used as one of a profile of tools to assess other important outcomes, including quality of life (QOL) or HRQL.

We identified two disease-specific measures developed specifically for patients with DR—the Diabetic Retinopathy Dependent Quality of Life (RetDQoL) and the Diabetic Retinopathy Treatment Satisfaction Questionnaire (RetTSQ). The tools have been developed in parallel, and to date, are the only measures that assess the impact of DR on different aspects of QOL. Unlike other tools identified in this review, the RetDQoL and RetTSQ have been designed to enable patients to consider specifically the impact of diabetic eye problems and their treatment, rather than health generally, vision or vision loss, or impact of diabetes.[18] Preliminary psychometric testing appears promising for content validity and reliability. Additional testing is ongoing to assess responsiveness and interpretability.

Despite the availability of reliable and valid tools to measure HRQL,[20,28,35] our review identified several studies that used questions or tools whose psychometric properties had not been evaluated. In order to provide meaningful HRQL data, it is crucial that the measurement tools are reliable, valid, and responsive (i.e., sensitive to change). In this way, researchers, clinicians, and patients will be better able to assess and interpret the impact of different interventions for DR on HRQL outcomes.

Impact of interventions on HRQL

To date, two RCTs have reported HRQL outcomes.[42,47] More are expected as a search of Clinicaltrails.gov identified 13 ongoing or recently completed trials investigating interventions for DME or DR that indicate the intention to report HRQL outcomes. The PKC-DRS2 trial of once-daily ruboxistaurin versus placebo measured HRQL using the SF–36 and the VFQ–25;[75] however, results for the HRQL outcomes have not been reported. Furthermore preliminary results from the RISE and RIDE trials[79] comparing ranibizumab versus sham have been presented at national meetings; however, to date, the final results for HRQL have not been published.

In general, it appears that HRQL outcomes improve following various interventions to treat DR at different levels of severity. For anti-VEGF to treat patients with DME, two RCTs with unclear risk of bias found statistically significant improvements in some domains of the VFQ–25; however, the results were not consistent at 1 year post-treatment. We concluded that the strength of evidence was low.

For other interventions, the results are based on one or two observational studies with a high risk of bias. Therefore, we conclude that the strength of evidence is insufficient to draw any conclusions about which of these interventions for DR are effective in improving HRQL. Furthermore, there is a concern about the applicability of the results of the observational studies to patients in North America. All of these studies were conducted in Europe or Japan. In particular, the three studies that were based in Japan used the Japanese version of the VFQ–25.

This review shows that the impact of interventions for DR on HRQL has not been adequately assessed in the current literature. Research has increasingly highlighted HRQL as an important health outcome in diabetes.[35] Diabetic patients with retinopathy have reported that vision loss impacts multiple areas of well-being including: independence, mobility, leisure, and self-care.[7,17,18] However, the impact is due not only to impaired vision, but also the emotional reaction to diagnosis and treatment, anxiety about the future, and advice to restrict physical activities.[18] For researchers and clinicians conducting trials of interventions for DR, the inclusion of HRQL outcomes will provide a better understanding how DR and its treatment affects outcomes that are important to patients.

Recommendations for Future Research

- RCTs are needed to assess the effectiveness of interventions for DR, including DME to improve HRQL. All RCTs investigating the effectiveness of interventions for DR should measure and report pre- and post-treatment HRQL outcomes.

- Currently, there are a number of ongoing or recently completed trials that reported the intention to capture HRQL outcomes. Future systematic reviews should followup on these studies and incorporate their findings, if appropriate.
- Researchers should use valid and reliable HRQL tools whose psychometric properties have been evaluated and reported.
- Ongoing assessment of psychometric properties of the DR specific tools is encouraged.
- Patients should be followed for at least 6 months post-intervention in order to capture maximum improvement for visual acuity.
- Use standard protocols to assess visual acuity to allow for comparison across trials
- RCTs should be designed and conducted to minimize risk of bias where at all possible. Authors may find tools such as the CONSORT[18,80] statement helpful in designing and reporting on RCTs.

Conclusions

We identified four HRQL measurement instruments that have been used to assess the impact of treatment in patients with DR. The psychometric properties of these tools have been adequately evaluated. Two tools developed specifically for patients with DR are currently undergoing evaluation. In general, HRQL was improved following interventions for DR and DME. Further research on HRQL following anti-VEGF treatment for DME is needed to confirm the results of two RCTs. The current research on the impact of other interventions for DR on HRQL is insufficient to draw conclusions about the relative effect of one intervention versus another. RCTs that assess the impact of treatments for DR should include HRQL as an outcome.

References

1. Congdon N, O'Colmain B, Klaver CC, et al. Causes and prevalence of visual impairment among adults in the United States. Arch Ophthalmol 2004;122(4):477-85.

2. Zhang X, Saaddine JB, Chou CF, et al. Prevalence of diabetic retinopathy in the United States, 2005-2008. JAMA 2010;304(6):649-56.

3. Saaddine JB, Honeycutt AA, Narayan KMV, et al. Projection of diabetic retinopathy and other major eye diseases among people with diabetes mellitus: United States, 2005-2050. Arch Ophthalmol 2008;126(12):1740-7.

4. The effect of intensive treatment of diabetes on the development and progression of long-term complications in insulin-dependent diabetes mellitus. The Diabetes Control and Complications Trial Research Group. N Engl J Med 1993;329(14):977-86.

5. Matthews DR, Stratton IM, Aldington SJ, et al. Risks of progression of retinopathy and vision loss related to tight blood pressure control in type 2 diabetes mellitus: UKPDS 69. Arch Ophthalmol 2004;122(11):1631-40.

6. Fong DS, Ferris FL, III, Davis MD, et al. Causes of severe visual loss in the early treatment diabetic retinopathy study: ETDRS report no. 24. Early Treatment Diabetic Retinopathy Study Research Group. Am J Ophthalmol 1999;127(2):137-41.

7. Javitt JC, Aiello LP. Cost-effectiveness of detecting and treating diabetic retinopathy. Ann Intern Med 1996;124(1:Pt 2):t-9.

8. American Academy of Opthalmology Retina Panel. Preferred practice pattern: diabetic retinopathy. 2008.

9. American Diabetes Association. Standards of Medical Care in Diabetes--2011. Diabetes Care 2011;34(Suppl 1):S11-S61.

10. American Optometric Association. Comprehensive adult eye and vision examination. 2005;2nd.

11. Vijan S, Hofer TP, Hayward RA. Cost-utility analysis of screening intervals for diabetic retinopathy in patients with type 2 diabetes mellitus. JAMA 2000;283(7):889-96.

12. Photocoagulation for diabetic macular edema. Early Treatment Diabetic Retinopathy Study report number 1. Early Treatment Diabetic Retinopathy Study research group. Arch Ophthalmol 1985;103(12):1796-806.

13. Photocoagulation for diabetic macular edema: Early Treatment Diabetic Retinopathy Study Report no. 4. The Early Treatment Diabetic Retinopathy Study Research Group. Int Ophthalmol Clin 1987;27(4):265-72.

14. Flynn HW, Jr., Chew EY, Simons BD, et al. Pars plana vitrectomy in the Early Treatment Diabetic Retinopathy Study. ETDRS report number 17. The Early Treatment Diabetic Retinopathy Study Research Group. Ophthalmology 1992;99(9):1351-7.

15. Nguyen QD, Shah SM, Khwaja AA, et al. Two-year outcomes of the ranibizumab for edema of the mAcula in diabetes (READ-2) study. Ophthalmology 2010;117(11):2146-51.

16. Preliminary report on effects of photocoagulation therapy. The Diabetic Retinopathy Study Research Group. Am J Ophthalmol 1976;81(4):383-96.

17. Coyne KS, Margolis MK, Kennedy-Martin T, et al. The impact of diabetic retinopathy: perspectives from patient focus groups. Family Practice 2004;21(4):447-53.

18. Woodcock A, Bradley C, Plowright R, et al. The influence of diabetic retinopathy on quality of life: interviews to guide the design of a condition-specific, individualised questionnaire: the RetDQoL. Patient Educ Couns 2004;53(3):365-83.

19. Sharma S, Oliver-Fernandez A, Bakal J, et al. Utilities associated with diabetic retinopathy: results from a Canadian sample. Evidence-Based Eye Care 2003;4(3):172-3.

20. Sharma S, Oliver-Fernandez A, Liu W, et al. The impact of diabetic retinopathy on health-related quality of life. [Review] [22 refs]. Curr Opin Ophthalmol 2005;16(3):155-9.

21. Baiardini I, Bousquet PJ, Brzoza Z, et al. Recommendations for assessing patient-reported outcomes and health-related quality of life in clinical trials on allergy: a GA(2)LEN taskforce position paper. Allergy 2010;65(3):290-5.

22. Patrick DL, Burke LB, Powers JH, et al. Patient-reported outcomes to support medical product labeling claims: FDA perspective. Value Health 2007;10 Suppl 2:S125-S137.

23. Guyatt GH, Feeny DH, Patrick DL. Measuring health-related quality of life. Ann Intern Med 1993;118(8):622-9.

24. Patrick DL, Bergner M. Measurement of health status in the 1990s. Annu Rev Public Health 1990;11:165-83.

25. Revicki DA, Osoba D, Fairclough D, et al. Recommendations on health-related quality of life research to support labeling and promotional claims in the United States. Qual Life Res 2000;9(8):887-900.

26. Higginson IJ, Carr AL, Robinson PG. Quality of Life. London: BMJ Books; 2003.

27. McDowell I, Newell C. The theoretical and technical foundations of health measurement. In: Measuring health, a guide to rating scales and questionnaires. Third ed. New York: Oxford Scholarship Online; 2006.

28. de Boer MR, Moll AC, de Vet HC, et al. Psychometric properties of vision-related quality of life questionnaires: a systematic review. Ophthalmic Physiol Opt 2004;24(4):257-73.

29. Mokkink LB, Terwee CB, Patrick DL, et al. The COSMIN study reached international consensus on taxonomy, terminology, and definitions of measurement properties for health-related patient-reported outcomes. J Clin Epidemiol 2010;63(7):737-45.

30. Assessing health status and quality-of-life instruments: attributes and review criteria. Qual Life Res 2002;11(3):193-205.

31. Hays RD, Anderson R, Revicki D. Psychometric considerations in evaluating health-related quality of life measures. Qual Life Res 1993;2(6):441-9.

32. Johnson D, Hollands S, Hollands H, et al. Quality of life amongst American vs. Canadian patients with retinal diseases. Curr Opin Ophthalmol 2010;21(3):227-32.

33. Lopes De Jesus CC, Atallah AN, Valente O, et al. Pentoxifylline for diabetic retinopathy. Cochrane Database of Systematic Reviews (2), 2008 Article Number: CD006693 Date of Publication: 2008 2008;(2).

34. O'Doherty M, Dooley I, Hickey-Dwyer M. Interventions for diabetic macular oedema: a systematic review of the literature. [Review] [60 refs]. Br J Ophthalmol 2008;92(12):1581-90.

35. Speight J, Reaney MD, Barnard KD. Not all roads lead to Rome - A review of quality of life measurement in adults with diabetes. Diabet Med 2009;26(4):315-27.

36. Mokkink LB, Terwee CB, Knol DL, et al. The COSMIN checklist for evaluating the methodological quality of studies on measurement properties: a clarification of its content. BMC Med Res Methodol 2010;10:22.

37. Albers G, Echteld MA, de Vet HC, et al. Evaluation of quality-of-life measures for use in palliative care: a systematic review. Palliat Med 2010;24(1):17-37.

38. Higgins J, Green S, eds. Cochrane handbook for systematic reviews of interventions. 5.1.0 ed. The Cochrane Collaboration; 2011.

39. Wells GA, Shea B, O'Connel D, et al. The Newcastle-Ottawa Scale (NOS) for assessing the quality of nonrandomized studies in meta-analysis. Department of Epidemiology and Community Medicine, University of Ottawa, Canada. 2011. Available from: URL: http://www.ohri.ca/programs/clinical_epidemiology/oxford.asp.

40. Owens DK, Lohr KN, Atkins D, et al. Grading the strength of a body of evidence when comparing medical interventions. Agency for Healthcare Research and Quality. 2008. [Accessed: 2010 Apr 21]; Available from: URL: http://www.effectivehealthcare.ahrq.gov/repFiles/2009_0805_grading.pdf.

41. Okamoto F, Okamoto Y, Fukuda S, et al. Vision-related quality of life and visual function after vitrectomy for various vitreoretinal disorders. Invest Ophthalmol Vis Sci 2010;51(2):744-51.

42. Sultan MB, Zhou D, Loftus J, et al. A phase 2/3, multicenter, randomized, double-masked, 2-year trial of pegaptanib sodium for the treatment of diabetic macular edema. Ophthalmology 2011;118(6):1107-18.

43. Okamoto F, Okamoto Y, Fukuda S, et al. Vision-related quality of life and visual function following vitrectomy for proliferative diabetic retinopathy. Am J Ophthalmol 2008;145(6):1031-6.

44. Loftus JV, Sultan MB, Pleil AM, et al. Changes in vision- and health-related quality of life in patients with diabetic macular edema treated with pegaptanib sodium or sham. Invest Ophthalmol Vis Sci 2011;52(10):7498-505.

45. Emi K, Oyagi T, Ikeda T, et al. [Influence of vitrectomy for diabetic retinopathy on health-related quality of life]. [Japanese]. Nippon Ganka Gakkai Zasshi 2008;112(2):141-7.

46. Emi K, Ikeda T, Bando H, et al. [Efficacy of treatments on vision-related quality of life in patients with diabetic retinopathy]. [Japanese]. Nippon Ganka Gakkai Zasshi 2009;113(11):1092-7.

47. Mitchell P, Bandello F, Schmidt-Erfurth U, et al. The RESTORE study: ranibizumab monotherapy or combined with laser versus laser monotherapy for diabetic macular edema. Ophthalmology 2011;118(4):615-25.

48. Tranos PG, Topouzis F, Stangos NT, et al. Effect of laser photocoagulation treatment for diabetic macular oedema on patient's vision-related quality of life. Current Eye Research 2004;29(1):41-9.

49. Matza LS, Rousculp MD, Malley K, et al. The longitudinal link between visual acuity and health-related quality of life in patients with diabetic retinopathy. HEALTH QUAL LIFE OUTCOMES 2008;6:95.

50. Boisjoly H, Gresset J, Charest M, et al. The VF-14 index of visual function in recipients of a corneal graft: a 2-year follow-up study. Am J Ophthalmol 2002;134(2):166-71.

51. Mozaffarieh M, Heinzl H, Sacu S, et al. Second eye cataract surgery in the diabetes patient? Quality of life gains and speed of visual and functional rehabilitation. Ophthalmic Research 2009;41(1):2-8.

52. Hernaez-Ortega MC, Soto-Pedre E, Pinies JA. Lanreotide Autogel for persistent diabetic macular edema. DIABETES RES CLIN PRACT 2008;80(3):e8-10.

53. Mozaffarieh M, Heinzl H, Sacu S, et al. Clinical outcomes of phacoemulsification cataract surgery in diabetes patients: visual function (VF-14), visual acuity and patient satisfaction. Acta Ophthalmol Scand 2005;83(2):176-83.

54. Mozaffarieh M, Benesch T, Sacu S, et al. Photocoagulation for diabetic retinopathy: determinants of patient satisfaction and the patient-provider relationship. Acta Ophthalmol Scand 2005;83(3):316-21.

55. Scanlon PH, Martin ML, Bailey C, et al. Reported symptoms and quality-of-life impacts in patients having laser treatment for sight-threatening diabetic retinopathy. Diabet Med 2006;23(1):60-6.

56. Ware JE, Jr., Sherbourne CD. The MOS 36-item short-form health survey (SF-36). I. Conceptual framework and item selection. Med Care 1992;30(6):473-83.

57. McHorney CA, Ware JE, Jr., Lu JF, et al. The MOS 36-item Short-Form Health Survey (SF-36): III. Tests of data quality, scaling assumptions, and reliability across diverse patient groups. Med Care 1994;32(1):40-66.

58. Stucki G, Liang MH, Phillips C, et al. The Short Form-36 is preferable to the SIP as a generic health status measure in patients undergoing elective total hip arthroplasty. Arthritis Care Res 1995;8(3):174-81.

59. Brazier JE, Harper R, Jones NM, et al. Validating the SF-36 health survey questionnaire: new outcome measure for primary care. BMJ 1992;305(6846):160-4.

60. Andresen EM, Patrick DL, Carter WB, et al. Comparing the performance of health status measures for healthy older adults. J Am Geriatr Soc 1995;43(9):1030-4.

61. Lyons RA, Perry HM, Littlepage BN. Evidence for the validity of the Short-form 36 Questionnaire (SF-36) in an elderly population. Age Ageing 1994;23(3):182-4.

62. Hayes V, Morris J, Wolfe C, et al. The SF-36 health survey questionnaire: is it suitable for use with older adults? Age Ageing 1995;24(2):120-5.

63. Mangione CM, Lee PP, Gutierrez PR, et al. Development of the 25-item National Eye Institute Visual Function Questionnaire. Arch Ophthalmol 2001;119(7):1050-8.

64. Klein R, Moss SE, Klein BE, et al. The NEI-VFQ-25 in people with long-term type 1 diabetes mellitus: the Wisconsin Epidemiologic Study of Diabetic Retinopathy. Arch Ophthalmol 2001;119(5):733-40.

65. Suzukamo Y, Oshika T, Yuzawa M, et al. Psychometric properties of the 25-item National Eye Institute Visual Function Questionnaire (NEI VFQ-25), Japanese version. HEALTH QUAL LIFE OUTCOMES 2005;3:65.

66. Steinberg EP, Tielsch JM, Schein OD, et al. The VF-14. An index of functional impairment in patients with cataract. Arch Ophthalmol 1994;112(5):630-8.

67. Bradley C. Diabetes treatment satisfaction questionnaire (DTSQ). In: Bradley C, ed. Handbook of psychology and diabetes: a guide to psychological measurement in diabetes research and management. New York: Psychology Press, Taylor & Francis Group; 1994:111-32.

68. Bradley C, Speight J. Patient perceptions of diabetes and diabetes therapy: assessing quality of life. Diabetes Metab Res Rev 2002;18 Suppl 3:S64-S69.

69. Bradley C, Todd C, Gorton T, et al. The development of an individualized questionnaire measure of perceived impact of diabetes on quality of life: the ADDQoL. Qual Life Res 1999;8(1-2):79-91.

70. Brose LS, Bradley C. Psychometric development of the individualized Retinopathy-Dependent Quality of Life questionnaire (RetDQoL). Value Health 2010;13(1):119-27.

71. Brose LS, Bradley C. Psychometric development of the retinopathy treatment satisfaction questionnaire (RetTSQ). Psychology Health & Medicine 2009;14(6):740-54.

72. Ware JE, Jr., Gandek B. Overview of the SF-36 Health Survey and the International Quality of Life Assessment (IQOLA) Project. J Clin Epidemiol 1998;51(11):903-12.

73. Mangione CM, Lee PP, Pitts J, et al. Psychometric properties of the National Eye Institute Visual Function Questionnaire (NEI-VFQ). NEI-VFQ Field Test Investigators. Arch Ophthalmol 1998;116(11):1496-504.

74. Cassard SD, Patrick DL, Damiano AM, et al. Reproducibility and responsiveness of the VF-14. An index of functional impairment in patients with cataracts. Arch Ophthalmol 1995;113(12):1508-13.

75. Lewis KS, Bradley C, Knight G, et al. A measure of treatment satisfaction designed specifically for people with insulin-dependent diabetes. Diabet Med 1988;5(3):235-42.

76. Horsman J, Furlong W, Feeny D, et al. The Health Utilities Index (HUI): concepts, measurement properties and applications. HEALTH QUAL LIFE OUTCOMES 2003;1:54.

77. Kaplan SH, Greenfield S, Ware JE, Jr. Assessing the effects of physician-patient interactions on the outcomes of chronic disease. Med Care 1989;27(3 Suppl):S110-S127.

78. Sherbourne CD, Hays RD, Ordway L, et al. Antecedents of adherence to medical recommendations: results from the Medical Outcomes Study. J Behav Med 1992;15(5):447-68.

79. Nguyen QD, Brown DM, Marcus DM, et al. Ranibizumab for Diabetic Macular Edema: Results from 2 Phase III Randomized Trials: RISE and RIDE. Ophthalmology 2012;119(4):789-801.

80. Schulz KF, Altman DG, Moher D. CONSORT 2010 statement: updated guidelines for reporting parallel group randomised trials. PLoS Med 2010;7(3):e1000251.

81. Woodcock A, Plowright R, Kennedy-Martin T, et al. Development of the new retinopathy treatment satisfaction questionnaire (RetTSQ). International Congress Series 2005;1282, 342-6.

Abbreviations and Acronyms

95% CI	95% confidence intervals
ADVS	Activities of Daily Vision Scale
BVCA	best corrected visual acuity
CONSORT	Consolidated Standards of Reporting Trials
COSMIN	COnsensus-based Standards for the selection of health Measurement Instruments
DME	diabetic macular edema
DR	diabetic retinopathy
DTSQ	Diabetic Treatment Satisfaction Questionnaire
dx	diagnosis
ETDRS	Early Treatment of Diabetic Retinopathy Study
HRQL	health-related quality of life
ICC	interclass correlation coefficient
logMAR	logarithm of minimal angle of resolution
MCS	mental component summary
MD	mean differences
mo	month
MOS	Medical Outcomes Study
NOS	Newcastle-Ottawa Scale
NPDR	nonproliferative diabetic retinopathy
NRCT	nonrandomized controlled trial
PCS	physical component summary
PDR	proliferative diabetic retinopathy
PRO	patient reported outcomes
Pt	patient
QOL	quality of life
RCT	randomized controlled trial
RetTSQ	Diabetic Retinopathy Treatment Satisfaction Questionnaire
RetDQoL	Diabetic Retinopathy Dependent Quality of Life
SES	socioeconomic status
SF–36	Short-Form Health Survey 36
SIP	Sickness Impact Profile
tx	treatment
UK	United Kingdom
US	United States
VA	visual acuity
VF	visual function
VF–14	Visual Function–14
VFQ–25	National Eye Institute Visual Function Questionnaire–25
yr	year

Appendices

Appendix A. Search strategies
Appendix B. Inclusion/exclusion form
Appendix C. List of excluded studies
Appendix D. Summary table of included HRQL assessment tools
Appendix E. Sample HRQL assessment tools
Appendix F. Extended study characteristics and outcomes for studies reporting the impact of interventions for diabetic retinopathy on HRQL

Appendix A. Search Strategies

Database: Ovid MEDLINE® <1950 to July 2010>

Search Strategy:
----

1   exp diabetes mellitus/
2   exp hyperinsulinism/
3   exp hypoglycemia/
4   exp hyperglycemia/
5   exp glycosuria/
6   diabet$.tw
7   mellitus.tw
8   ((non insulin adj depend$ adj3 diabetes mellitus) OR (noninsulin$ adj depend$ adj3 diabetes mellitus)).tw.
9   ((insulin adj depend$ adj3 diabetes mellitus) OR (insulindepend$ adj3 diabetes mellitus)).tw.
10   ((type 1 OR type I) adj2 (diabetes mellitus OR DM)).tw
11   ((type 2 OR type II) adj2 (diabetes mellitus OR DM)).tw
12   (T1DM OR T2DM OR ((T1 OR T2) adj DM)).tw
13   ((maturity OR late) adj onset adj diabet$).tw
14   IDDM.tw
15   NIDDM.tw
16   MODY.tw
17   DM.tw
18   OR/1-17 (392,571)
19   exp vision disORders/
20   exp diabetic retinopathy/
21   exp retinal detachment/
22   exp retinal degeneration/
23   exp retinal hemORrhage/
24   exp retinal neovascularization/
25   exp retinal vein occlusion/
26   exp epiretinal membrane/
27   exp vitreORetinopathy, proliferative/
28   exp vitreous detachment/
29   exp vitreous hemORrhage/
30   exp macular edema/
31   (eye disease$ OR blindness OR visual loss$).tw
32   (vis$ adj funct$).tw
33   (retinopath$ OR retinitis OR maculopath$).tw
34   (diabet$ adj3 maculopath$).tw
35   macula$ adj $edema.tw
36   macula$ adj (defect$ OR degenerat$ OR swell$).tw
37   microaneurysm$.tw
38   neovascular$.tw
39   OR/19-38 (142,484)
40   18 AND 39 (23,376)
41   exp "quality of life"/
42   exp quality-adjusted life years/
43   exp health status/
44   exp health status indicatORs/
45   exp "value of life"/
46   exp self concept/
47   exp "activities of daily living"/
48   exp "severity of illness index"/
49   exp sickness impact profile/

50 exp patient satisfaction/
51 exp questionnaires/
52 "quality of life".tw
53 "health related quality of life".tw
54 (health adj status).tw
55 (QoL OR QL).tw
56 QALY.tw
57 HRQL.tw
58 (life adj3 qualit$).tw
59 (funct$ adj (assess$ OR abilit$)).tw
60 "patient repORted outcomes".tw
61 ADL$.tw
62 OR/41-61 (607,847)
63 SF?36.tw
64 SF?12.tw
65 EuroQol.tw
66 "Quality of Well-Being".tw
67 "National Eye Institute Visual Functioning Questionnaire".tw
68 "Visual Function Index".tw
69 "Activities of Daily Vision".tw
70 "Daily Living Tasks Dependent on Vision".tw
71 "sickness impact profile".tw
72 RAND?36.tw
73 RAND?12.tw
74 "health utilities index".tw
75 "quality of well-being scale".tw
76 "standard gamble".tw
77 "time-trade off".tw
78 WHO-BREF.tw
79 "diabetes health profile".tw
80 "diabetes quality of life".tw
81 "diabetes quality of life clinical trial questionnaire".tw
82 "well-being questionnaire".tw
83 OR 63-82 (4,196)
84 exp depression/
85 exp anxiety/
86 exp anxiety disORders/
87 exp mental disORders/
88 exp mental health/
89 exp mental fatigue/
90 exp stress, psychological/
91 exp social behaviOR/
92 "life stress".tw
93 anxiet*.tw
94 depress*.tw
95 nervous*.tw
96 (coping adj2 strateg*).tw
97 psychosocial*.tw
98 psychological*.tw
99 (mental adj health).tw
100 (social adj2 (skill* OR behavi?OR)).tw
101 OR/84-100 (1,352,438)
102 62 OR 83 OR 101 (1,789,878)
103 40 AND 102 (1,731)

Database: Ovid EMBASE® <1980 to July 2010>

Search Strategy:
----

1. exp diabetes mellitus/
2. exp hyperinsulinism/
3. exp hypoglycemia/
4. exp hyperglycemia/
5. exp glycosuria/
6. diabet$.tw
7. mellitus.tw
8. ((non insulin adj depend$ adj diabetes mellitus) OR (noninsulin$ adj depend$ adj diabetes mellitus)).tw.
9. (insulin adj depend$ adj diabetes mellitus).tw.
10. ((type 1 OR type I) adj (diabetes mellitus OR DM)).tw
11. ((type 2 OR type II) adj (diabetes mellitus OR DM)).tw
12. (T1DM OR T2DM OR ((T1 OR T2) adj DM)).tw
13. ((maturity OR late) adj onset adj diabet$).tw
14. IDDM.tw
15. NIDDM.tw
16. MODY.tw
17. DM.tw
18. OR/1-17 (508,740)
19. exp visual disORder/
20. exp diabetic retinopathy/
21. exp retina detachment/
22. exp retina degeneration/
23. exp retina hemORrhage/
24. exp retinal neovascularization/
25. exp retinal vein occlusion/
26. exp vitreORetinopathy
27. exp vitreous body detachment/
28. exp vitreous hemORrhage/
29. (eye disease$ OR blindness OR visual loss$).tw
30. (vis$ adj funct$).tw
31. (retinopath$ OR retinitis OR maculopath$).tw
32. macula$ adj $edema.tw
33. macula$ adj (defect$ OR degenerat$ OR swell$).tw
34. microaneurysm$.tw
35. neovascular$.tw
36. OR/19-35 (270,247)
37. 18 AND 36 (33,026)
38. exp "quality of life"/
39. exp quality adjusted life year/
40. exp health status/
41. exp health survey/
42. exp self concept/
43. exp daily life activity/
44. exp Sickness Impact Profile/
45. exp patient satisfaction/
46. exp questionnaire/
47. "quality of life".tw
48. "health related quality of life".tw
49. (health adj status).tw
50. (QoL OR QL).tw
51. QALY.tw
52. HRQL.tw

53 (life adj3 qualit$).tw
54 (funct$ adj (assess$ OR abilit$)).tw
55 "patient repORted outcomes".tw
56 ADL$.tw
57 health status indicatOR$.tw
58 value of life.tw
59 act$ of daily living.tw
60 (severity adj3 (illness index OR disease index)).tw
61 OR/38-60 (465,498)
62 exp ShORt FORm36/
63 exp ShORt FORm12.tw
64 exp National Eye Institute Visual Functioning Questionnaire/
65 EuroQol.tw
66 quality of well-being.tw
67 visual function index.tw
68 activities of daily vision.tw
69 daily living tasks dependent on vision.tw
70 RAND-36.tw
71 RAND-12.tw
72 health utilities index.tw
73 quality of well-being scale.tw
74 standard gamble.tw
75 time-trade off.tw
76 WHO-BREF.tw
77 diabetes health profile.tw
78 diabetes quality of life.tw
79 diabetes quality of life clinical trial questionnaire.tw
80 well-being questionnaire.tw
81 OR/62-80 (9,399)
82 exp depression/
83 exp anxiety/
84 exp anxiety disORders/
85 exp mental health/
86 exp life stress/
87 exp coping behaviOR/
88 depress$.tw
89 anxiety$.tw
90 nervous$.tw
91 (coping adj2 strateg$).tw
92 psychosocial$.tw
93 psychological$.tw
94 (mental adj health).tw
95 (social adj2 (skill$ OR behavi?OR)).tw
96 OR/82-95 (793,003)
97 61 OR 81 OR 96 (1,396,857)
98 37 AND 97 (2,979)

Database: Ovid PsychINFO <1806 to July 2010>
Search Strategy:

1	exp diabetes mellitus/
2	exp hypoglycemia/
3	exp hyperglycemia/
4	diabet$.tw
5	mellitus.tw
6	((non insulin adj depend$ adj3 diabetes mellitus) OR (noninsulin$ adj depend$ adj3 diabetes mellitus)).tw.
7	(insulin adj depend$ adj3 diabetes mellitus).tw.
8	((type 1 OR type I) adj2 (diabetes mellitus OR DM)).tw
9	((type 2 OR type II) adj2 (diabetes mellitus OR DM)).tw
10	(T1DM OR T2DM OR ((T1 OR T2) adj DM)).tw
11	((maturity OR late) adj onset adj diabet$).tw
12	IDDM.tw
13	NIDDM.tw
14	MODY.tw
15	DM.tw
16	hyperinsulinism.tw
17	glycosuria.tw
18	OR/1-17 (13,235)
19	exp vision disORders/
20	(eye disease$ OR blindness OR visual loss$).tw
21	(vis$ adj funct$).tw
22	(retinopath$ OR retinitis OR maculopath$).tw
23	(diabet$ adj3 maculopath$).tw
24	macula$ adj $edema.tw
25	macula$ adj (defect$ OR degenerat$ OR swell$).tw
26	microaneurysm$.tw
27	neovascular$.tw
28	(diabet$ adj3 retinopath$).tw
29	(retina$ adj3 detach$).tw
30	(retina$ adj3 degenerat$).tw
31	(retina$ adj3 h$emORrhage).tw
32	(retina$ adj3 neovasculari*ation).tw
33	(retina$ adj3 vein occlusion).tw
34	epiretinal membrane.tw
35	vitreORetinopathy.tw
36	(vitreous adj3 (detach$ OR h?emORrhage)).tw
37	OR/19-36 (17,045)
38	18 AND 37 (323)
39	exp "quality of life"/
40	exp life satisfaction/
41	exp self concept/
42	exp "activities of daily living"/
43	exp client satisfaction/
44	exp questionnaires/
45	"quality of life".tw
46	"health related quality of life".tw
47	(health adj status).tw
48	(QoL OR QL).tw
49	QALY.tw
50	HRQL.tw
51	(life adj3 qualit$).tw

52	(funct$ adj (assess$ OR abilit$)).tw
53	"patient repORted outcomes".tw
54	ADL$.tw
55	(health adj3 (status OR status indicatOR$)).tw
56	value of life.tw
57	(severity adj3 (illness index OR disease index)).tw
58	sickness impact profile.tw
59	OR/39-58 (116,240)
60	SF–36.tw
61	SF–12.tw
62	EuroQol.tw
63	Quality of Well-Being.tw
64	National Eye Institute Visual Functioning Questionnaire.tw
65	Visual Function Index.tw
66	Daily Living Tasks Dependent on Vision.tw
67	RAND-36.tw
68	RAND-12.tw
69	health utilities index.tw
70	quality of well-being scale.tw
71	standard gamble.tw
72	time-trade off.tw
73	WHO-BREF.tw
74	diabetes health profile.tw
75	diabetes quality of life.tw
76	diabetes quality of life clinical trial questionnaire.tw
77	well-being questionnaire.tw
78	OR 60-77 (3,135)
79	59 OR 78 (116,961)
80	exp majOR depression/
81	exp anxiety/
82	exp anxiety disORders/
83	exp mental health/
84	exp mental disORders/
85	exp stress, psychological/
86	exp coping behaviOR/
87	"life stress".tw
88	anxiet*.tw
89	depress*.tw
90	nervous*.tw
91	(coping adj2 strateg*).tw
92	psychosocial*.tw
93	psychological*.tw
94	(mental adj health).tw
95	(social adj2 (skill* OR behavi?OR)).tw
96	OR/80-95 (795,694)
97	79 OR 96 (866,765)
98	38 AND 97 (113)

Database: Ovid Cochrane Central Register of Control Trials <1991 to July 2010>

Search Strategy:
----
1 exp diabetes mellitus/
2 exp hyperinsulinism/
3 exp hypoglycemia/
4 exp hyperglycemia/
5 exp glycosuria/
6 diabet$.tw
7 mellitus.tw
8 ((non insulin adj depend$ adj3 diabetes mellitus) OR (noninsulin$ adj depend$ adj3 diabetes mellitus)).tw.
9 (insulin adj depend$ adj3 diabetes mellitus).tw.
10 ((type 1 OR type I) adj2 (diabetes mellitus OR DM)).tw
11 ((type 2 OR type II) adj2 (diabetes mellitus OR DM)).tw
12 (T1DM OR T2DM OR ((T1 OR T2) adj DM)).tw
13 ((maturity OR late) adj onset adj diabet$).tw
14 IDDM.tw
15 NIDDM.tw
16 MODY.tw
17 DM.tw
18 OR/1-17 (21,104)
19 exp vision disORders/
20 exp diabetic retinopathy/
21 exp retinal detachment/
22 exp retinal degeneration/
23 exp retinal hemORrhage/
24 exp retinal neovascularization/
25 exp retinal vein occlusion/
26 exp epiretinal membrane/
27 exp vitreORetinopathy, proliferative/
28 exp vitreous detachment/
29 exp vitreous hemORrhage/
30 exp macular edema/
31 (eye disease$ OR blindness OR visual loss$).tw
32 (vis$ adj funct$).tw
33 (retinopath$ OR retinitis OR maculopath$).tw
34 (diabet$ adj3 maculopath$).tw
35 macula$ adj $edema.tw
36 macula$ adj (defect$ OR degenerat$ OR swell$).tw
37 microaneurysm$.tw
38 neovascular$.tw
39 OR/19-38 (4,902)
40 18 AND 39 (1,377)
41 exp "quality of life"/
42 exp quality-adjusted life years/
43 exp health status/
44 exp health status indicatORs/
45 exp "value of life"/
46 exp self concept/
47 exp "activities of daily living"/
48 exp "severity of illness index"/
49 exp sickness impact profile/
50 exp patient satisfaction/

51 exp questionnaires/
52 "quality of life".tw
53 "health related quality of life".tw
54 (health adj status).tw
55 (QoL OR QL).tw
56 QALY.tw
57 HRQL.tw
58 (funct$ adj (assess$ OR abilit$)).tw
59 "patient repORted outcomes".tw
60 ADL$.tw
61 OR/41-61 (44,357)
62 SF–36.tw
63 SF–12.tw
64 EuroQol.tw
65 "Quality of Well-Being".tw
66 "National Eye Institute Visual Functioning Questionnaire".tw
67 "Visual Function Index".tw
68 "Activities of Daily Vision".tw
69 Daily Living Tasks Dependent on Vision.tw
70 sickness impact profile.tw
71 RAND-36.tw
72 health utilities index.tw
73 quality of well-being scale.tw
74 standard gamble.tw
75 time-trade off.tw
76 WHO-BREF.tw
77 diabetes health profile.tw
78 diabetes quality of life.tw
79 diabetes quality of life clinical trial questionnaire.tw
80 well-being questionnaire.tw
81 OR/62-80 (2,457)
82 62 OR 81 (44,449)
83 exp depression/
84 exp anxiety/
85 exp anxiety disORders/
86 exp mental disORders/
87 exp mental health/
88 exp mental fatigue/
89 exp stress, psychological/
90 exp social behaviOR/
91 "life stress".tw
92 anxiet*.tw
93 depress*.tw
94 nervous*.tw
95 (coping adj2 strateg*).tw
96 psychosocial*.tw
97 psychological*.tw
98 (mental adj health).tw
99 (social adj2 (skill* OR behavi?OR)).tw
100 OR/93-99 (64,320)
101 82 OR 100 (96,404)
102 40 AND 101 (71)

Database: CINAHL Plus with full text <1937 to July 2010>

Search Strategy:

S108=S46 AND S107 (1,651)
S107=S67 OR S88 OR S106 (593,052)
S106=S89 OR S90 OR S91 OR S92 OR S93 OR S94 OR S95 OR S96 OR S97 OR S98 OR S99 OR S100 OR S101 OR S102 OR S103 OR S104 OR S105 (552,364)
S105=TX coping N2 strateg*
S104=TX social N2 behavi#OR
S103=TX social N2 skill*
S102=TX mental N1 health
S101=TX psychological*
S100=TX psychosocial*
S99=TX nervous*
S98=TX depress*
S97=TX anxiet*
S96=TX "life stress"
S95=TX "life stress"
S94=MH "Social BehaviOR+"
S93=MH "Stress, Psychological+"
S92=MH "Mental Health"
S91=MH "Mental DisORders+"
S90=MH "Anxiety DisORders+"
S89=MH "Anxiety+"
S88=S68 OR S69 OR S70 OR S71 OR S72 OR S73 OR S74 OR S75 OR S76 OR S77 OR S78 OR S79 OR S80 OR S81 OR S82 OR S83 OR S84 OR S85 OR S86 OR S87 (33,010)
S87=TX "well-being questionnaire"
S86=TX "diabetes quality of life clinical trial questionnaire"
S85=TX "diabetes quality of life"
S84=TX "diabetes health profile"
S83=TX WHO-BREF
S82=TX "time-trade off"
S81=TX "standard gamble"
S80=TX "quality of well-being scale"
S79=TX" health utilities index"
S78=TX RAND#12
S77=TX RAND#36
S76=TX "sickness impact profile"
S75= TX "activities of daily vision"
S74= TX "visual function index"
S73=TX "national eye institute visual functioning questionnaire"
S72=TX "quality of well-being"
S71=TX EuroQoL
S70=TX sf#12
S69=TX sf#36
S68=MH "Severity of Illness Indices+"
S67=S47 OR S48 OR S49 OR S50 OR S51 OR S52 OR S53 OR S54 OR S55 OR S56 OR S57 OR S58 OR S59 OR S60 OR S61 OR S62 OR S63 OR S64 OR S65 OR S66 (310,508)
S66=TX ADL*
S65=TX "patient reported outcomes"
S64=TX (funct* N1 assess*) OR (funct* abilit*)
S63=TX life N3 qualit*
S62=TX HRQL

S61=TX QALY
S60=TX QoL
S59=TX (health N1 status)
S58=TX "health related quality of life"
S57=TX "quality of life"
S56=MH "Questionnaires+"
S55=MH "Patient Satisfaction"
S54=MH "Sickness Impact Profile"
S53=MH "Severity of Illness"
S52=MH "Activities of Daily Living+"
S51=MH "Self Concept+"
S50=MH "Health Status IndicatORs"
S49=MH "Health Status+"
S48=MH "Quality-Adjusted Life Years"
S47=MH "Quality of Life+"
S46=S21 AND S45 (4,823)
S45=S22 OR S23 OR S24 OR S25 OR S26 OR S27 OR S28 OR S29 OR S30 OR S31 OR S32 OR S33 OR S34 OR S35 OR S36 OR S37 OR S38 OR S39 OR S40 OR S41 OR S42 OR S43 OR S44 (19,362)
S44=TX vitreous h#emORrhage
S43=TX vitreous detach*
S42=TX vitreORetinopathy
S41=TX epiretinal membrane
S40=TX retina* N1 neovasculari?ation
S39=TX retina* N1 vein occlusion
S38=TX retina* N1 detach*
S37=TX retina* N1 degenerat*
S36=TX microaneurysm*
S35=TX neovascular*
S34=TX macula* N1 swell*
S33=TX macula* N1 degenerat*
S32=TX macula* N1 defect*
S31=TX macula* N1 #edema
S30=TX (diabet* N3 maculopath*)
S29=TX (retinopath* OR blindness OR visual loss*)
S28=TX (vis* N1 funct*)
S27=TX (eye disease* OR blindeness OR visual loss*)
S26=MH "Retinal Diseases+"
S25=MH "Eye HemORrhage"
S24=MH "Retinal Detachment"
S23=MH "Diabetic Retinopathy"
S22=MH "Vision DisORders+"
S21=S1 OR S2 OR S3 OR S4 OR S5 OR S6 OR S7 OR S8 OR S9 OR S10 OR S11 OR S12 OR S13 OR S14 OR S15 OR S16 OR S17 OR S18 OR S19 OR S20 (161,039)
S20=TX DM
S19=TX MODY
S18=TX NIDDM
S17=TX IDDM
S16=TX ((maturity onset N2 diabet*) OR (late onset N2 diabet*))
S15=TX (T1 N1 DM) OR (T2 N1 DM)
S14=TX (T1DM OR T2DM)
S13=TX (type II N2 diabetes mellitus) OR (type II N2 DM)
S12=TX (type 2 N2 diabetes mellitus) OR (type 2 N2 DM)
S11=TX (type I N2 diabetes mellitus) OR (type I N2 DM)
S10=TX ((type 1 N2 diabetes mellitus) OR (type 1 N2 DM))
S9=TX (insulin N1 depend* N3 diabetes mellitus)
S8=TX ((non insulin N1 depend* N3 diabetes mellitus) OR (noninsulin* N1 depend* N3 diabetes mellitus))

S7=TX mellitus
S6=TX diabet*
S5=TX glycosuria
S4=MH Hypoglycemia+
S3=MH Hyperglycemia+
S2=MH Hyperinsulinism+
S1=MH Diabetes Mellitus+

Database: Scopus <1823 to July 2010>
Search Strategy:

((TITLE-ABS-KEY("diabetes PRE/1 mellitus") OR (diabet*) OR (mellitus)) AND (TITLE-ABS-KEY("diabetic PRE/1 retinopath*") OR (blindness) OR ("visual PRE/1 loss*") OR ("vis* PRE/1 funct*") OR (retinopath*) OR (retinitis) OR (maculopath*) OR ("macula* PRE/1 defect*") OR ("macula* PRE/1 degenerat*") OR ("macula* PRE/1 swell*")) AND ((TITLE-ABS-KEY("quality PRE/1 life") OR ("health PRE/1 status") OR ("value PRE/1 life") OR ("self PRE/1 concept") OR ("activities PRE/1 daily living") OR ("sickness impact profile") OR ("patient PRE/1 satisfaction") OR ("patient PRE/1 repORted outcome*")) OR (TITLE-ABS-KEY(depression) OR (anxiety) OR ("anxiety PRE/1 disORder*") OR ("mental PRE/1 disORder*") OR ("mental PRE/1 health") OR ("mental PRE/1 fatigue") OR ("coping PRE/1 strateg*")))) (1,244)

Database: Clinicaltrials.gov, Results <April 2011>

NCT Number	Title	Study Condition	Intervention	HRQL measure
NCT01131585	Safety and efficacy of ranibizumab in diabetic macular edema	Diabetic macular edema; proliferative diabetic retinopathy	Ranibizumab + laser; sham injections + laser	Unspecified QOL
NCT00701181	Prospective, randomized, multi-center, comparator study evaluating efficacy and safety of PF-04523655 versus laser in subjects with diabetic macular edema	Diabetic retinopathy; diabetes complications	Laser treatment; PF-04523655 (high dose); PF-04523655 (middle dose); PF-04523655 (low dose)	VFQ–25
NCT00090519	Reduction in the occurrence of center-involved diabetic macular edema	Diabetic retinopathy	Ruboxistaurin; placebo	VFQ–25
NCT00799227	Safety and efficacy of a new treatment in vitrectomized subjects with diabetic macular edema	Diabetic macular edema	Dexamethasone	VFQ–25
NCT00464685	Safety and efficacy of a new treatment in combination with laser for diabetic macular edema	Diabetic macular edema	Dexamethasone; sham injection	Unspecified QOL
NCT00168389	A study of the safety and efficacy of a new treatment for diabetic macular edema	Diabetic macular edema	Dexamethasone; sham dexamethasone	Unspecified QOL
NCT01171976	Efficacy and safety of Ranibizumab in two "treat and extend" treatment algorithms versus Ranibizumab as needed in patients with	Diabetic macular edema	Ranibizumab	VFQ-25

	macular edema and visual impairment secondary to diabetes mellitus (RETAIN)			
NCT00473382	A study of ranibizumab injection in subjects with clinically significant macular edema with center involvement secondary to diabetes mellitus (RIDE)	Diabetes mellitus macular edema	Ranibizumab; sham	VFQ–25
NCT00473330	A study of ranibizumab injection in subjects with clinically significant macular edema with center involvement secondary to diabetes mellitus (RISE)	Diabetes mellitus macular edema	Ranibizumab; sham	VFQ–25
NCT00989989	Efficacy and Safety of Ranibizumab (Intravitreal Injections) in Patients With Visual Impairment Due to Diabetic Macular Edema	Diabetic macular edema	Ranibizumab; Laser photocoagulation	Unspecified PROs
NCT01292798	Treatment of Residual Diabetic Macular Edema With Ranibizumab	Diabetic macular edema	Ranibizumab	Participant scores on unspecified work productivity and activity impairment questionnaire
NCT01318941	Observe the effectiveness and safety of Ranibizumab in real life setting	Wet age-related macular degeneration, diabetic macular edema, retinal vein occlusion	Ranibizumab	VFQ–25
NCT01331681	VEGF Trap-Eye in vision impairment due to diabetic macular edema (DME)	Diabetes mellitus; macular edema	VEGF Trap-Eye (BAY86-5321); VEGF Trap-Eye (BAY86-5321); Laser treatment	Unspecified QOL

Appendix B. Inclusion/Exclusion Form

	Reviewer ID	Ref ID
	Criteria	**Decision**
1.	**Report of Primary Research**	☐ Yes ☐ No ☐ Unsure
2.	**Population:** Adults (≥18 years)	☐ Yes ☐ No ☐ Unsure
3.	**Population:** Diagnosed with diabetic retinopathy or diabetic macular edema or neovascular	☐ Yes ☐ No ☐ Unsure
4a.	**Measurement:** Does the study report on the use of a patient-reported HRQL measure (physical, social, emotional, mental function)?	☐ Yes ☐ No ☐ Unsure
4b.	**Measurement:** Does the study report on the use of a patient-reported HRQL measure (physical, social, emotional, mental function) in the context of assessing an intervention (with or without a comparator) for DR?	☐ Yes ☐ No ☐ Unsure
	Reviewer Decision	☐ Yes ☐ No ☐ Unsure
	CONSENSUS DECISION	☐ INCLUDE ☐ EXCLUDE

*Flag studies that do not investigate an intervention for DR, but do provide the psychometric properties of a HRQL tool.

☐ Abstract requiring full publication	
☐ Requires translation	Specify source language

Appendix C. Excluded Studies

482 studies were excluded from the review. Reasons for exclusion include: publication type (n=78), age being less than 18 years (n=3), diagnosis without DR (n=117), intervention (n=99), outcomes (n=185).

Publication type (n = 78)

1. Diabetic retinopathy on a new scale. J Am Optom Assoc 2003;74(11):735-8.

2. The aging retina: diseases of the retina. Insight 2007;1(4):2-15.

3. Assessing care of vulnerable elders-3 quality indicators. J Am Geriatr Soc 2007;55(Suppl):87.

4. Ophthalmic inserts shown to improve dry eye symptoms, quality of life. Ocular Surgery News 2009;27(11):20.

5. Abbaszadeh AS, Tabatabaei MO, Pajouhi M. Diabetes in old age, a review. Iran J Diabetes Lipid Disord 2009;8(1):113-28.

6. Averbukh E, Banin E. Diabetic macular edema: towards therapy aimed at the underlying pathogenic mechanisms. Isr Med Assoc J 2006;8(2):127-8.

7. Baker RS. Diabetic retinopathy in African Americans: vision impairment, prevalence, incidence, and risk factors. Int Ophthalmol Clin 2003;43(4):105-22.

8. Balcer LJ. Optic neuritis. New Engl J Med 2006;354(12):1273-80.

9. Bernstein RK. Depression in adults with diabetes. Diabetes Care 1993;16(5):847-8.

10. Brown CM, Wong EYH, O'Connor PM, et al. Measurement of quality of life for people with diabetic retinopathy impairment. Expert Rev Ophthalmol 2009;4(6):587-93.

11. Caditz J. An education-support-group program for visually impaired people with diabetes. J Vis Impairm Blindn 1992;86(1):81-3.

12. Carney C. Diabetes mellitus and major depressive disorder: an overview of prevalence, complications, and treatment. Depress Anxiety 1998;7(4):149-57.

13. Cheah JS, Lim P. Diabetic retinopathy and metabolic control. Ann Acad Med Singapore 1980;9(1):104-6.

14. Cherner R. Help for the sight-impaired diabetic patient. Consultant (00107069) 1997;37(4):916-8.

15. Cherner R. Primary care update. Help for the sight-impaired diabetic patient. Consultant (00107069) 1997;37(4):916-8.

16. Chew EY. A simplified diabetic retinopathy scale. Ophthalmology 2003;110(9):1675-6.

17. Chipkin SR, Klugh SA, Chasan-Taber L. Exercise and diabetes. Cardiol Clin 2001;19(3):489-505.

18. Cleary ME. Aiding the person who is visually impaired from diabetes. Diabetes Educ 1985;10(4):12-23.

19. Consoli A, Gomis R, Halimi S, et al. Initiating oral glucose-lowering therapy with metformin in type 2 diabetic patients: an evidence-based strategy to reduce the burden of late-developing diabetes complications. Diabetes Metab 2004;30(6):509-16.

20. Dineen B, Waldron-Lynch F, Harney F, et al. Laser photocoagulation for diabetic retinopathy. Cochrane Database of Syst Rev 2008;(1):CD006960.

21. Donohue B, Acierno R, Hersen M, et al. Social skills training for depressed, visually impaired older adults. A treatment manual. Behav Modif 1995;19(4):379-424.

22. Eastman R. Cost-effectiveness of detecting and treating diabetic retinopathy... commentary on Javitt JC and Aiello L. Ann Intern Med 124:164-9, 1996. Diabetes Spectr 1996;9(3):182-3.

23. Falavarjani KG, Modarres M, Nazari H, et al. Diabetic macular edema following panretinal photocoagulation. Arch Ophthalmol 2010;128(2):262.

24. Fenwick EK, Pesudovs K, Rees G, et al. The impact of diabetic retinopathy: understanding the patient's perspective. [Review]. Br J Ophthalmol 2011;95(6):774-82.

25. Frank RN. Importance of the NHANES 2005-2008 diabetic: Retinopathy data. Arch Ophthalmol 2011;(6):June.

26. Gardner TW. The restore study: Ranibizumab monotherapy or combined with laser versus laser monotherapy for diabetic macular edema. Evidence-Based Ophthalmology 2011;(4):October.

27. Garg MK, Baliga KV. Management of type 2 diabetes (NIDDM). Med J Armed Forces India 2002;58(1):53-9.

28. Gill G. Psychological aspects of diabetes. Br J Hosp Med 1991;46(5):301-5.

29. Gillibrand W, Holdich P. Evidence-based management 20 assessment of retinopathy. Pract Nurs 2010;21(6):305-9.

30. Gonder-Frederick LA, Cox DJ, Ritterband LM. Diabetes and behavioral medicine: the second decade. J Consult Clin Psychol 2002;70(3):611-25.

31. Graham C, Lasko-McCarthey P. Exercise options for persons with diabetic complications. Diabetes Educ 1990;16(3):212-20.

32. Grigorian RA, Castellarin A, Bhagat N, et al. Use of viscodissection and silicone oil in vitrectomy for severe diabetic retinopathy. Semin Ophthalmol 2003;18(3):121-6.

33. Guerra CE, Datto CJ, Kim KH, et al. Quality of life instrument and retinal diseases. Ophthalmology 2004;111(3):608-9.

34. Harper-Jaques S. Diabetes under control: diabetes and depression. Am J Nurs 2004;104(9):56-9.

35. Hart J. Diabetes and complementary therapies: research review and clinical applications. Altern Complement Therap 2006;12(6):263-7.

36. Henzen C. The diabetic--a difficult patient difficult to treat? Praxis 2006;95(14):541-4.

37. Herpertz S, Petrak F, Albus C, et al. Evidence-based diabetes guidelines of the German diabetes society: psychosocial factors and diabetes mellitus. Diabetes Stoffwechsel 2003;12(1):35-58.

38. Horowitz A. Depression and vision and hearing impairments in later life. Generations 2003;27(1):32-8.

39. Horowitz A, Reinhardt JP. Adequacy of the mental health system in meeting the needs of adults who are visually impaired. J Vis Impair Blind 2006;100(Suppl.):871-4.

40. Jacobson AM. The psychological care of patients with insulin-dependent diabetes mellitus. New Engl J Med 1996;334(19):1249-53.

41. Jindal K, MacNair L, Senior P. A collaborative approach to diabetes nephropathy prevention. Alberta RN 2005;61(9):10-1.

42. Katon WJ. The comorbidity of diabetes mellitus and depression. Am J Med 2008;121(11):Suppl. 2.

43. Kieffer KM, Reese RJ. A reliability generalization study of the geriatric depression scale. Educ Psychol Meas 2002;62(6):969-94.

44. Mendrinos E, Donati G, Pournaras CJ. Rapid and persistent regression of severe new vessels on the disc in proliferative diabetic retinopathy after a single intravitreal injection of pegaptanib. Acta Opthalmologica 2009;87(6):683-4.

45. Merrill JL. Support groups for persons with diabetes and visual impairment. J Vis Impair Blind 1993;87(9):376-7.

46. Montez JK, Karner TX. Understanding the diabetic body-self. Qual Health Res 2005;15(8):1086-104.

47. Norris SL. Health-related quality of life among adults with diabetes. Curr Diabetes Rep 2005;5(2):124-30.

48. Norris SL, Kansagara D, Bougatsos C, et al. Screening adults for type 2 diabetes: A review of the evidence for the U.S. preventive services task force. Ann Intern Med 2008;148(11):855-68.

49. Oehler-Giarratana J. Meeting the psychosocial and rehabilitative needs of the visually impaired diabetic. J Vis Impair Blind 1978;72(9):358-61.

50. Orr AL, Huebner KM. Toward a collaborative working relationship among vision rehabilitation and allied health professionals. J Vis Impair Blind 2001;95(8):468-82.

51. Orticio LP. Measuring health-related quality of life among older visually impaired adults: a preview to instrument construction. Insight 2007;32(3):8-12.

52. Paulus YM, Gariano RF. Diabetic retinopathy: a growing concern in an aging population. Geriatrics 2009;64(2):16-20.

53. Pompei P. Diabetes mellitus in later life. Generations 2006;30(3):39-44.

54. Porta M, Bandello F. Diabetic retinopathy: a clinical update. Diabetologia 2002;45(12):1617-34.

55. Pouwer F, Hermanns N. Insulin therapy and quality of life. A review. Diabetes Metab Res Rev 2009;25(Suppl. 1)

56. Prasad S. Survey of diabetic retinopathy screening services in England and Wales. Diabet Med 1999;16(3):269.

57. Rao PM. Diabetic retinopathy: new proposed classification. Indian J Ophthalmol 2008;56(5):440-1.

58. Raphael BA, Galetta KM, Jacobs DA. Validation and test characteristics of a 10-item neuro-ophthalmic supplement to the NEI-VFQ-25. Rev Neurol Dis 2007;4(4):234.

59. Robertson C. Coping with chronic complications... diabetes. RN 1989;52(9):34.

60. Rosenthal AR. Failing sight. Br Med J 1990;301(6745):244.

61. Rosenthal MJ. Analyses of nursing home residents with diabetes at admission. J Am Med Dir Assoc 2004;5(5):353-5.

62. Rubin RR, Ciechanowski P, Egede LE, et al. Recognizing and treating depression in patients with diabetes. Curr Diabetes Rep 2004;4(2):119-25.

63. Sahu AK, Majji AB. Effect of ruboxistaurin on the visual acuity decline associated with long-standing diabetic macular edema. Invest Ophthalmol Vis Sci 2010;51(12):6890-1.

64. Servat JJ, Risco M, Nakasato YR, et al. Visual impairment in the elderly: Impact on functional ability and quality of life. Clin Geriatr 2011;19(7):49-56.

65. Shotliff K, Balasanthiran A. Diabetic retinopathy and eye screening. Pract Nurs 2009;38(9):23.

66. Smiddy WE, Flynn J. Vitrectomy in the management of diabetic retinopathy. Surv Ophthalmol 1999;43(6):491-507.

67. Sokol-McKay D, Buskirk K, Whittaker P. Adaptive low-vision and blindness techniques for blood glucose monitoring. Diabetes Educ 2003;29(4):614-8.

68. Strachan MWJ. Fear of diabetes complications. Diabetes Metab Res Rev 2005;21(3):262-3.

69. Taylor HR. Diabetic retinopathy. Clin Exp Ophthalmol 2005;33(1):3-4.

70. Ting JH, Martin DK. Basic and clinical aspects of gene therapy for retinopathy induced by diabetes. Curr Gene Ther 2006;6(2):193-214.

71. Torrance GW. Utility approach to measuring health-related quality of life. J Chronic Dis 1987;40(6):593-603.

72. Van Den Bosch-De Haeselaer. Quality of life of the diabetic. Louvain Med 2003;122(9):S308-S313.

73. Vijan S, Hofer TP, Hayward RA. Cost-utility analysis of screening intervals for diabetic retinopathy in patients with type 2 diabetes mellitus. Clin Cornerstone 2001;4(2):65.

74. Williams AS, Ponchillia SV. Psychosocial sequelae of visual loss in diabetes. Diabetes Educ 1998;24(6):675-6.

75. Wroe J. Spring 2005 Meeting of the Association of British Clinical Diabetologists. Pract Diabetes Int 2005;22(7):272-274a.

76. Yamada Y, Takasawa T, Hirasawa Y, et al. Vision rehabilitation for the once-sighted blind report 5-Present condition and problems in communication and activities of daily living. Folia Ophthalmol Jpn 1999;50(9):687-91.

77. Yospaiboon Y, Ratanapakorn T. Pars plana vitrectomy for diabetic macular edema. Cochrane Database of Syst Rev 2007;(2):CD006126.

78. Zhang HW, Zhang H, Wan X, et al. Herbal medicine for diabetic retinopathy. Cochrane Database of Syst Rev 2009;(3):CD007939.

Age <18 yr (n = 3)

1. Hassan K, Loar R, Anderson BJ, et al. The role of socioeconomic status, depression, quality of life, and glycemic control in type 1 diabetes mellitus. J Pediatr 2006;149(4):526-31.

2. Nicolucci A, Maione A, Franciosi M, et al. Quality of life and treatment satisfaction in adults with Type 1 diabetes: A comparison between continuous subcutaneous insulin infusion and multiple daily injections. Diabet Med 2008;25(2):213-20.

3. Strohmeier SM, Back M, Egger JW, et al. Expectations concerning future life and late complications by adolescents and young adults with type 1 diabetes. Diabetes Stoffwechsel 1998;7(6):233-7.

Diagnosis without DR (n = 117)

1. Leads from the MMWR. Improving eye care for persons with diabetes mellitus--Michigan. JAMA 1985 Dec 20;254(23):3293-4.

2. Influence of intensive diabetes treatment on quality-of-life outcomes in the diabetes control and complications trial. Diabetes Care 1996 Mar;19(3):195-203.

3. In brief. Program helps relieve distress of age-related eye disease. Harvard Women's Health Watch 2005 Jun;12(10):7.

4. Abramoff MD, Suttorp-Schulten MS. Web-based screening for diabetic retinopathy in a primary care population: the EyeCheck project. Telemedicine Journal & E-Health 2005 Dec;11(6):668-74.

5. Ahmadian L, Massof R. Does functional vision behave differently in low-vision patients with diabetic retinopathy?--A case-matched study. Invest Ophthalmol Vis Sci 2008 Sep;49(9):4051-7.

6. Alabraba V, Farnsworth A, Leigh R, Dodson P, et al. Exubera inhaled insulin in patients with type 1 and type 2 diabetes: the first 12 months. Diabetes Technol Ther 2009 Jul;11(7):427-30.

7. Allen EM, Ziada HM, O'Halloran D, Clerehugh V, et al. Attitudes, awareness and oral health-related quality of life in patients with diabetes. J Oral Rehabil 2008 Mar;35(3):218-23.

8. Bergh AL, Persson LO, Attvall S. Psychometric properties of the Swedish version of the Well +ó-Being Questionnaire in a sample of patients with diabetes type 1. Scand J Public Health 2000;28(2):137-45.

9. Bonanomi MT, Nicoletti AG, Carricondo PC, Buzalaf F, et al. Retinal thickness assessed by optical coherence tomography (OCT) in pseudophakic macular edema. Arq Bras Oftalmol 2006 Jul;69(4):539-44.

10. Bond GE, Burr RL, Wolf FM, Feldt K. The effects of a web-based intervention on psychosocial well-being among adults aged 60 and older with diabetes: A randomized trial. Diabetes Educ 2010;36(3):446-56.

11. Brandle M, Davidson MB, Schriger DL, Lorber B, et al. Cost effectiveness of statin therapy for the primary prevention of major coronary events in individuals with type 2 diabetes. Diabetes Care 2003 Jun;26(6):1796-801.

12. Broman AT, Munoz B, Rodriguez J, Sanchez R, et al. The impact of visual impairment and eye disease on vision-related quality of life in a Mexican-American population: proyecto VER. Invest Ophthalmol Vis Sci 2002 Nov;43(11):3393-8.

13. Cacciatore F, Abete P, Maggi S, Luchetti G, et al. Disability and 6-year mortality in elderly population. Role of visual impairment. Aging Clin Exp Res 2004 Oct;16(5):382-8.

14. Camacho F, Anderson RT, Bell RA, Goff J, et al. Investigating correlates of health related quality of life in a low-income sample of patients with diabetes. Qual Life Res 2002;11(8):783-96.

15. Chen JY, Diamant AL, Thind A, Maly RC. Determinants of breast cancer knowledge among newly diagnosed, low-income, medically underserved women with breast cancer. Cancer 2008;112(5):1153-61.

16. Chia E-M, Wang JJ, Rochtchina E, Smith W, et al. Impact of bilateral visual impairment on health-related quality of life: the Blue Mountains Eye Study. Invest Ophthalmol Vis Sci 2004 Jan;45(1):71-6.

17. Claiborne N, Massaro E. Mental quality of life: an indicator of unmet needs in patients with diabetes. Soc Work Health Care 2000;32(1):25-43.

18. Clarke P, Gray A, Holman R. Estimating utility values for health states of type 2 diabetic patients using the EQ-5D (UKPDS 62). Med Decis Mak 2002 Jul;22(4):340-9.

19. Clarke PM, Simon J, Cull CA, Holman RR. Assessing the impact of visual acuity on quality of life in individuals with type 2 diabetes using the short form-36. Diabetes Care 2006 Jul;29(7):1506-11.

20. Crewe JM, Morlet N, Morgan WH, et al. Quality of life of the most severely vision-impaired. Clin Exp Ophthalmol 2011;39(4):336-43.

21. Covic AM, Iyengar SK, Olson JM, Sehgal AR, et al. A family-based strategy to identify genes for diabetic nephropathy. Am J Kidney Dis 2001 Mar;37(3):638-47.

22. Dreer LE, Berry J, Rivera P, Snow M, et al. Efficient assessment of social problem-solving abilities in medical and rehabilitation settings: a Rasch analysis of the Social Problem-Solving Inventory-Revised. J Clin Psychol 2009 Jul;65(7):653-69.

23. Echeverry D, Duran P, Bonds C, Lee M, et al. Effect of pharmacological treatment of depression on A1C and quality of life in low-income hispanics and African Americans with diabetes: A randomized, double-blind, placebo-controlled trial. Diabetes Care 2009;32(12):2156-60.

24. Espinet LM, Osmick MJ, Ahmed T, Villagra VG. A cohort study of the impact of a national disease management program on HEDIS diabetes outcomes. Disease Management 2005 Apr;8(2):86-92.

25. Frost NA, Sparrow JM, Durant JS, Donovan JL, et al. Development of a questionnaire for measurement of vision-related quality of life. Ophthalmic Epidemiol 1998;5(4):185-210.

26. Gillibrand W. Users' perception of a mobile diabetic eye-screening service. J Diabetes Nurs 2000 May;4(3):82-5.

27. Glasgow RE, Nutting PA, King DK, Nelson CC, et al. A practical randomized trial to improve diabetes care. J Gen Intern Med 2004 Dec;19(12):1167-74.

28. Gulliford MC, Mahabir D. Relationship of health-related quality of life to symptom severity in diabetes mellitus: A study in Trinidad and Tobago. J Clin Epidemiol 1999;52(8):773-80.

29. Hahm BJ, Shin YW, Shim EJ, Jeon HJ, et al. Depression and the vision-related quality of life in patients with retinitis pigmentosa. Br J Ophthalmol 2008;92(5):650-4.

30. Hawthorne G. Assessing utility where short measures are required: Development of the short assessment of quality of life-8 (AQoL-8) Instrument. Value Health 2009 Sep;12(6):948-57.

31. Hill-Briggs F, Gary TL, Hill MN, Bone LR, et al. Health-related quality of life in urban African Americans with type 2 diabetes. J Gen Int Med 2002;17(6):412-9.

32. Holbrook EA, Caputo JL, Perry TL, Fuller DK, et al. Physical activity, body composition, and perceived quality of life of adults with visual impairments. J Vis Impair Blind 2009;103(1):17-29.

33. Holmes J, Mcgill S, Kind P, Bottomley J, et al. Health-related quality of life in type 2 diabetes. Value Health 2000;3(Suppl. 1):S47-S51.

34. Huang F, Yang Q, Chen L, Tang S, et al. Renal pathological change in patients with type 2 diabetes is not always diabetic nephropathy: a report of 52 cases. Clinical Nephrology 2007 May;67(5):293-7.

35. Huang GH, Palta M, Allen C, LeCaire T, et al. Self-rated health among young people with type 1 diabetes in relation to risk factors in a longitudinal study. Am J Epidemiol 2004 Feb 15;159(4):364-72.

36. Inoue A. Visual disability due to diabetic nephropathy and its effect on quality of life in patients on maintenance hemodialysis. Folia Ophthalmol Jpn 2000;51(3):297-301.

37. Jennings DL, Ragucci KR, Chumney ECG, Wessell AM. Impact of clinical pharmacist intervention on diabetes related quality-of-life in an ambulatory care clinic. Pharmacy Practice 2007 Nov;5(4):169-73.

38. Ji YH, Park HJ, Oh SY. Clinical effect of low vision aids. Korean J Ophthalmol 1999 Jun;13(1):52-6.

39. Johnson JA, Maddigan SL. Performance of the RAND-12 and SF–12 summary scores in type 2 diabetes. Qual Life Res 2004;13(2):449-56.

40. Jung CS, Bruce B, Newman NJ, Biousse V. Visual function in anterior ischemic optic neuropathy: effect of Vision Restoration Therapy--a pilot study. J Neurol Sci 2008 May 15;268(1-2):145-9.

41. Kaholokula JK, Haynes SN, Grandinetti A, Chang HK. Ethnic differences in the relationship between depressive symptoms and health-related quality of life in people with type 2 diabetes. Ethnicity & Health 2006 Feb;11(1):59-80.

42. Kalter-Leibovici O, Wainstein J, Ziv A, Harman-Bohem I, et al. Clinical, socioeconomic, and lifestyle parameters associated with erectile dysfunction among diabetic men. Diabetes Care 2005 Jul;28(7):1739-44.

43. Kazis LE, Miller DR, Clark JA, Skinner KM, et al. Improving the response choices on the Veterans SF–36 Health Survey role functioning scales: results from the Veterans Health Study. Journal of Ambulatory Care Management 2004 Jul;27(3):263-80.

44. Kean-Cowdin R, Varma R, Wu J, Hays RD, et al. Severity of visual field loss and health-related quality of life. Am J Ophthalmol 2007;143(6):1013-23.

45. Keinanen-Kiukaanniemi S, Ohinmaa A, Pajunpaa H, Koivukangas P. Health related quality of life in diabetic patients measured by the Nottingham Health Profile. Diabet Med 1996 Apr;13(4):382-8.

46. Klein BE, Klein R, Moss SE. Self-rated health and diabetes of long duration. The Wisconsin Epidemiologic Study of Diabetic Retinopathy. Diabetes Care 1998 Feb;21(2):236-40.

47. Kodjebacheva G, Coleman AL, Ensrud KE, Cauley JA, et al. Reliability and Validity of Abbreviated Surveys Derived from the National Eye Institute Visual Function Questionnaire: The Study of Osteoporotic Fractures. Am J Ophthalmol 2010;149(2):330-40.

48. Kohara R, Hirao RA, Kitamura T, Kouhara H. Diabetes Conference: 69th Annual Meeting of the American Diabetes Association New Orleans, LA United States 2009.

49. Korkina MV, Elfimova EV. Diabetes mellitus and depression. Zh Nevrologii Psihiatrii im S S Korsakova 2003;103(12):66-70.

50. Labiris G, Katsanos A, Fanariotis M, Tsirouki T, et al. Psychometric properties of the Greek version of the NEI-VFQ 25. BMC Ophthalmol 2008;8.

51. Leas BF, Berman B, Kash KM, Crawford AG, et al. Quality measurement in diabetes care. Popul Heath Manage 2009 Oct;12(5):265-71.

52. Lee A. Knowledge provides the key to successful management of diabetic retinopathy. Ophthalmic Nurs 2000 Jun;4(1):12-6.

53. Lee PP, Whitcup SM, Hays RD, Spritzer K, et al. The relationship between visual acuity and functioning and well-being among diabetics. Qual Life Res 1995 Aug;4(4):319-23.

54. Lee PP, Spritzer K, Hays RD. The impact of blurred vision on functioning and well-being. Ophthalmology 1997 Mar;104(3):390-6.

55. Leksell J, Sandberg G, Wikblad K. Experiences of an educational programme for individuals with blindness caused by diabetes. European Diabetes Nursing 2006 Sep;3(2):86-91.

56. Li Y, Crews JE, Elam-Evans LD, et al. Visual impairment and health-related quality of life among elderly adults with age-related eye diseases. Qual Life Res 2011;20(6):845-52.

57. Lloyd CE, Matthews KA, Wing RR, Orchard TJ. Psychosocial factors and complications of IDDM. The Pittsburgh Epidemiology of Diabetes Complications Study. VIII. Diabetes Care 1992 Feb;15(2):166-72.

58. Lundman B, Asplund K, Norberg A. Living with diabetes: perceptions of well-being. Res Nurs Health 1990 Aug;13(4):255-62.

59. Ma SL, Shea JA, Galetta SL, Jacobs DA, et al. Self-reported visual dysfunction in multiple sclerosis: new data from the VFQ-25 and development of an MS-specific vision questionnaire. Am J Ophthalmol 2002 May;133(5):686-92.

60. Maahs DM, Gendelman N, Snell-Bergeon JK, McFann K, et al. Diabetes Conference: 69th Annual Meeting of the American Diabetes Association New Orleans, LA United States 2009.

61. Maddigan SL, Feeny DH, Johnson JA. Construct validity of the RAND-12 and Health Utilities Index Mark 2 and 3 in type 2 diabetes. Qual Life Res 2004;13(2):435-48.

62. Malik RA WSA. Effect of angiotensin-converting-enzyme (ACE) inhibitor trandolapril on human diabetic neuropathy: randomised double-blind controlled trial. Lancet 1998 Dec 19;(9145):1978-81.

63. Martinez-Castelao A, Gorriz JL, Garcia-Lopez F, Lopez-Revuelta K, et al. Perceived health-related quality of life and comorbidity in diabetic patients starting dialysis (CALVIDIA study). J Nephrol 2004;17(4):544-51.

64. Mason-Schrock D. Transsexuals' Narrative Construction of the "True Self". Soc Psychol Q 1996;59(3):176-92.

65. McCarty CA, McKay R, Keeffe JE. Management of diabetic retinopathy by Australian ophthalmologists. Working Group on Evaluation of the NHMRC Retinopathy Guideline Distribution. National Health and Medical Research Council. Clin Exp Ophthalmol 2000 Apr;28(2):107-12.

66. McCarty CA, Wright S, McKay R, Taylor KI, et al. Changes in management of diabetic retinopathy by Australian ophthalmologists as a result of the NHMRC clinical guidelines. Clin Exp Ophthal 2001 Aug;29(4):230-4.

67. McCarty CA, Taylor KI, McKay R, Keeffe JE, et al. Diabetic retinopathy: effects of national guidelines on the referral, examination and treatment practices of ophthalmologists and optometrists. Clin Exp Ophthal 2001 Apr;29(2):52-8.

68. McFarland KF, Rhoades DR, Campbell J, Finch WH. Meaning of illness and health outcomes in type 1 diabetes. Endocr Pract 2001 Jul;7(4):250-5.

69. McGill MJ, Molyneaux LM, O'Dea JA, Yue DK. Discussing diabetic retinopathy with NIDDM patients: An evaluation of varying the content of information given to patients and its impact on anxiety. Pract Diabetes Int 1995;12(4):173-6.

70. Mehta Z, Cull C, Stratton I, Yudkin J, et al. Quality of life in type 2 diabetic patients is affected by complications but not by intensive policies to improve blood glucose or blood pressure control (UKPDS 37). Diabetes Care 1999;22(7):1125-36.

71. Miljanovic B, Dana R, Sullivan DA, Schaumberg DA. Impact of dry eye syndrome on vision-related quality of life. Am J Ophthalmol 2007 Mar;143(3):409-15.

72. Misajon R, Hawthorne G, Richardson J, Barton J, et al. Vision and quality of life: The development of a utility measure. Invest Ophthalmol Vis Sci 2005;46(11):4007-15.

73. Miskala PH, Bressler NM, Meinert CL, Scott IU. Relative contributions of reduced vision and general health to NEI-VFQ scores in patients with neovascular age-related macular degeneration. Evid Based Eye Care 2004 Oct;5(4):222-3.

74. Mitchell J, Bradley C. Psychometric evaluation of the 12-item Well-being Questionnaire for use with people with macular disease. Qual Life Res 2001;10(5):465-73.

75. Mitchell J, Bradley C. Design of an individualised measure of the impact of macular disease on quality of life (the MacDQoL). Qual Life Res 2004 Aug;13(6):1163-75.

76. Mitchell J, Wolffsohn JS, Woodcock A, Anderson SJ, et al. +Psychometric evaluation of the MacDQoL individualised measure of the impact of macular degeneration on quality of life. Health Qual Life Outcomes 2005;3.

77. Mocan MC, Kadayifcilar S, Eldem B. Elevated intravitreal interleukin-6 levels in patients with proliferative diabetic retinopathy. Can J Ophthalmol 2006 Dec;41(6):747-52.

78. Mok JY, Laing IA, Farquhar JW. Young diabetics: memories, current lifestyles and attitudes. Diabet Med 1984 Sep;1(3):227-30.

79. Moon SH, Kim IH, Park SW, Kim I, et al. Early adjuvant radiotherapy toward long-term survival and better quality of life for craniopharyngiomas--a study in single institute. Childs Nervous System 2005 Aug;21(8-9):799-807.

80. Mozaffarieh M, Krepler K, Heinzl H, Sacu S, et al. Visual function, quality of life and patient satisfaction after ophthalmic surgery: a comparative study. Ophthalmologica 2004 Jan;218(1):26-30.

81. Nang EE, Khoo CM, Tai ES, Lim SC, et al. Is there a clear threshold for fasting plasma glucose that differentiates between those with and without neuropathy and chronic kidney disease?: the Singapore Prospective Study Program. Am J Epidemiol 2009 Jun 15;169(12):1454-62.

82. Nasser J, Habib F, Hasan M, Khalil N. Prevalence of depression among people with diabetes attending diabetes clinics at primary health settings. Bahrain Med Bull 2009 Sep;31(3).

83. Nirmalan PK, Tielsch JM, Katz J, Thulasiraj RD, et al. Relationship between vision impairment and eye disease to vision-specific quality of life and function in rural India: the Aravind Comprehensive Eye Survey. Invest Ophthalmol Vis Sci 2005 Jul;46(7):2308-12.

84. O'Connor PJ, Desai JR, Solberg LI, Rush WA, et al. Variation in diabetes care by age: opportunities for customization of care. BMC Fam Pract 2003 Oct 29;4:16.

85. Odin VI, Belikova TV, Pushkova ES. Diabetes mellitus in the elderly: succinic acid compounds in treating diabetic neuropathies. Adv Gerontol 2002;9:83-7.

86. Okamoto F, Okamoto Y, Hiraoka T, Oshika T. Vision-related Quality of Life and Visual Function after Retinal Detachment Surgery. Am J Ophthalmol 2008;146(1).

87. Okamoto F, Okamoto Y, Hiraoka T, Oshika T. Effect of Vitrectomy for Epiretinal Membrane on Visual Function and Vision-Related Quality of Life. Am J Ophthalmol 2009;147(5).

88. Olsen H, Jeune B, ndersen-Ranberg K. Centenarians in the county of Funen. Morbidity and functional capacity. Ugeskrift for Laeger 1996 Dec 16;158(51):7397-401.

89. Passamonti M, Pigni M, Colombo L, Sacchi E. The quality of life of patients with type 2 diabetes mellitus in general practice. Eur J Gen Pract 2000;6(3):93-7.

90. Raphael BA, Galetta KM, Jacobs DA, Markowitz CE, et al. Validation and test characteristics of a 10-item neuro-ophthalmic supplement to the NEI-VFQ–25. Am J Ophthalmol 2006 Dec;142(6):1026-35.

91. Reeves BC, Langham J, Walker J, Grieve R, et al. Verteporfin Photodynamic Therapy Cohort Study. Report 2: Clinical Measures of Vision and Health-Related Quality of Life. Ophthalmology 2009;116(12):2463-70.

92. Roh MI, Byeon SH, Kwon OW. Repeated intravitreal injection of bevacizumab for clinically significant diabetic macular edema. Retina 2008 Oct;28(9):1314-8.

93. Salive ME, Guralnik J, Christen W, Glynn RJ, et al. Functional blindness and visual impairment in older adults from three communities. Ophthalmology 1992 Dec;99(12):1840-7.

94. Savoia E, Fantini MP, Pandolfi PP, Dallolio L, et al. Assessing the construct validity of the Italian version of the EQ-5D: Preliminary results from a cross-sectional study in North Italy. Health Qual Life Outcomes 2006 Aug;4(47).

95. Schmid KL, Swann PG, Pedersen C, Schmid LM. The detection of diabetic retinopathy by Australian optometrists. Clin Exp Optometry 2002 Jul;85(4):221-8.

96. Sinclair AJ, Bayer AJ, Girling AJ, Woodhouse KW. Older adults, diabetes mellitus and visual acuity: a community-based case-control study. Age Ageing 2000 Jul;29(4):335-9.

97. Smith SC. Nursing interventions for ophthalmic patients with diabetes. Insight 2007 Oct;32(4):12-3.

98. Sousa VD, Zanetti ML, Zauszniewski JA, Mendes IAC, et al. Psychometric properties of the Portuguese version of the Depressive Cognition Scale in Brazilian adults with diabetes mellitus. Journal of Nursing Measurement 2008 Sep;16(2):125-35.

99. Stein JD, Brown MM, Brown GC, Hollands H, et al. Quality of life with macular degeneration: Perceptions of patients, clinicians and community members. Evid Based Eye Care 2003 Jul;4(3):176-8.

100. Steinberg EP, Tielsch JM, Schein OD, Javitt JC, et al. The VF–14. An index of functional impairment in patients with cataract. Arch Ophthalmol 1994 May;112(5):630-8.

101. Stelmack JA, Moran D, Dean D, Massof RW. Short- and long-term effects of an intensive inpatient vision rehabilitation program. Arch Phys Med Rehabil 2007 Jun;88(6):691-5.

102. Styles CJ, Park SJ, McGhee CN, Gamble G, et al. Evaluating the use of a scanning laser-derived oedema index to grade diabetic retinopathy and maculopathy. Clin Exp Ophthalmol 2007 Jan;35(1):18-23.

103. Sugawara T, Kaneko Y. Report of the second Iwate study trial on complications of diabetes mellitus - Questionnaire survey of patients attending the "DM Eye Seminar". Folia Ophthalmol Jpn 2004;55(3):197-201.

104. Sullivan P. Don't give up on GWAS. Mol Psychiatry 2011;(1):January.

105. Szlyk JP, Becker JE, Fishman GA, Seiple W. Psychological profiles of patients with central vision loss. J Vis Impair Blind 2001;95(1):781-6.

106. Talbot F, Nouwen A, Gingras J, B+®langer A, et al. Relations of diabetes intrusiveness and personal control to symptoms of depression among adults with diabetes. Health Psychol 1999;18(5):537-42.

107. Toprak AB, Eser E, Guler C, Baser FE, et al. Cross-validation of the Turkish version of the 25-item National Eye Institute Visual Functioning Questionnaire (NEI-VFQ 25). Ophthalmic Epidemiol 2005 Aug;12(4):259-69.

108. Tournier M, Moride Y, Ducruet T, Moshyk A, et al. Depression and mortality in the visually-impaired, community-dwelling, elderly population of Quebec. Acta Opthalmologica 2008 Mar;86(2):196-201.

109. Veen-de Vries NR, Luteijn AJ, Nasiiro RS, Meyboom-de JB. Health status of the elderly in the Marigot Health District, Dominica. West Indian Med J 1999 Jun;48(2):73-80.

110. Vileikyte L, Leventhal H, Gonzalez JS, Peyrot M, et al. Diabetic peripheral neuropathy and depressive symptoms: The association revisited. Diabetes Care 2005;28(10):2378-83.

111. Wills CJ, Scott A, Swift PG, Davies MJ, et al. Retrospective review of care and outcomes in young adults with type 1 diabetes. BMJ 2003 Aug 2;327(7409):260-1.

112. Wright SE, McKay R, Taylor KI, Keeffe JE, et al. Changes in attitudes and practices of optometrists in their management of diabetic retinopathy after the release of NHMRC guidelines. National Health and Medical Research Council. Clin Exp Ophthal 2001 Jun;29(3):121-4.

113. Yan S, Li Q, Sun YQ. Multivariate analysis of patients with diabetes mellitus accompanied by depression. Chin J Clin Rehab 2005;9(12):1-3.

114. Yang Z, Lin W, Moshfeghi DM, Thirumalaichary S, et al. A novel mutation in the RDS/Peripherin gene causes adult-onset foveomacular dystrophy. Am J Ophthalmol 2003 Feb;135(2):213-8.

115. Zhang CX, Chen YM, Chen WQ. Association of psychosocial factors with anxiety and depressive symptoms in Chinese patients with type 2 diabetes. Diabetes Res Clin Pract 2008;79(3):523-30.

116. Zhang X, Gregg EW, Cheng YJ, Thompson TJ, et al. Diabetes mellitus and visual impairment: national health and nutrition examination survey, 1999-2004. Arch Ophthalmol 2008 Oct;126(10):1421-7.

117. Zhou H, Isaman DJ, Messinger S, Brown MB, et al. A computer simulation model of diabetes progression, quality of life, and cost. Diabetes Care 2005 Dec;28(12):2856-63.

Intervention (n = 99)

1. Early worsening of diabetic retinopathy in the Diabetes Control and Complications Trial. Arch Ophthalmol 1998;116(7):874-86.

2. Alva ML, Gray A, Mihaylova B, et al. Diabetologia Conference: 46th Annual Meeting of the European Association for the Study of Diabetes, EASD 2010 Stockholm Sweden:S52.

3. Arai M. Low-vision care for rehabilitation of visually impaired due to diabetic retinopathy. Folia Ophthalmol Jpn 2005;56(5):311-5.

4. Awdeh RM, Elsing SH, Deramo VA, et al. Vision-related quality of life in persons with unilateral branch retinal vein occlusion using the 25-item National Eye Institute Visual Function Questionnaire. Br J Ophthalmol 2010;94(3):319-23.

5. Bamashmus MA, Gunaid AA, Khandekar R. Regular visits to a diabetes clinic were associated with lower magnitude of visual disability and diabetic retinopathy-a hospital-based historical cohort study in yemen. Diabetes Technol Ther 2009;11(1):45-50.

6. Bothe N, Hetzer R, Deinlein E. Patients with late-life vision damage in occupational rehabilitation. Preliminary ophthalmologic treatment, concomitant manifestations and an illustration provided by the growing number of patients with juvenile diabetes. Klin Monatsbl Augenheilkd 1992;200(1):1-4.

7. Brown MM, Brown GC, Sharma S, et al. Utility values and diabetic retinopathy. Am J Ophthalmol 1999;128(3):324-30.

8. Brown MM, Brown GC, Sharma S. Cost-effective analysis: Diabetic vitrectomy. Evidence-Based Eye Care 2001;2(2):117-21.

9. Brown MM, Brown GC, Sharma S, et al. Quality of life with visual acuity loss from diabetic retinopathy and age-related macular degeneration. Arch Ophthalmol 2002;120(4):481-4.

10. Byeon SH, Kwon OW, Song JH, et al. Prolongation of activity of single intravitreal bevacizumab by adjuvant topical aqueous depressant (Timolol-Dorzolamide). Graefes Arch Clin Exp Ophthalmol 2009;247(1):35-42.

11. Cha YJ, Kim SJ. The therapeutic effects of angiotensin-converting enzyme inhibitors in severe non-proliferative diabetic retinopathy. Korean J Ophthalmol 2007;21(1):28-32.

12. Chaturvedi N, Porta M, Klein R, et al. Effect of candesartan on prevention (DIRECT-Prevent 1) and progression (DIRECT-Protect 1) of retinopathy in type 1 diabetes: randomised, placebo-controlled trials. Lancet 2008;372(9647):1394-402.

13. Chew EY, Ferris FL, III, Csaky KG, et al. The long-term effects of laser photocoagulation treatment in patients with diabetic retinopathy: the early treatment diabetic retinopathy follow-up study. Ophthalmology 2003;110(9):1683-9.

14. Coffey JT, Brandle M, Zhou H, et al. Valuing health-related quality of life in diabetes. Diabetes Care 2002;25(12):2238-43.

15. Comty CM, Leonard A, Shapiro FL. Psychosocial problems in dialyzed diabetic patients. Kidney Int Suppl 1974;(1):144-51.

16. Coyne KS, Margolis MK, Kennedy-Martin T, et al. The impact of diabetic retinopathy: perspectives from patient focus groups. Fam Pract 2004;21(4):447-53.

17. Cusick M, SanGiovanni JP, Chew EY, et al. Central visual function and the NEI-VFQ-25 near and distance activities subscale scores in people with type 1 and 2 diabetes. Am J Ophthalmol 2005;139(6):1042-50.

18. Dasbach EJ, Klein R, Klein BE, et al. Self-rated health and mortality in people with diabetes. Am J Public Health 1994;84(11):1775-9.

19. Davidov E, Breitscheidel L, Clouth J, et al. Diabetic retinopathy and health-related quality of life. Graefes Arch Clin Exp Ophthalmol 2009;247(2):267-72.

20. Davis MD, Sheetz MJ, Aiello LP, et al. Effect of ruboxistaurin on the visual acuity decline associated with long-standing diabetic macular edema. Invest Ophthalmol Vis Sci 2009;50(1):1-4.

21. Diolaiuti S, Senn P, Schmid MK, et al. Combined pars plana vitrectomy and phacoemulsification with intraocular lens implantation in severe proliferative diabetic retinopathy. Ophthalmic Surg Lasers Imaging 2006;37(6):468-74.

22. Diskin CJ, Stokes TJ, Dansby LM, et al. A hypothesis: can erythropoietin administration affect the severity of retinopathy in diabetic patients with renal failure? Am J Med Sci 2007;334(4):260-4.

23. Dreer LE, Elliott TR, Berry J, et al. Cognitive appraisals, distress and disability among persons in low vision rehabilitation. Br J Health Psychol 2008;13(Pt:3):3-61.

24. el Haddad OA, Saad MK. Prevalence and risk factors for diabetic retinopathy among Omani diabetics. Br J Ophthalmol 1998;82(8):901-6.

25. Esteban JJ, Martinez MS, Navalon PG, et al. Visual impairment and quality of life: gender differences in the elderly in Cuenca, Spain. Qual Life Res 2008;17(1):37-45.

26. Ferguson SC, Blane A, Perros P, et al. Cognitive ability and brain structure in type 1 diabetes: relation to microangiopathy and preceding severe hypoglycemia. Diabetes 2003;52(1):149-56.

27. Fernandez GA, Sierra J, I. Analysis of eye disease and adaptation of visual aids in low vision patients: review of 1,000 cases. Arch Soc Esp Oftalmol 2001;76(9):527-32.

28. Finger RP, Kupitz DG, Holz FG, et al. The impact of the severity of vision loss on vision-related quality of life in india: An evaluation of the IND-VFQ-33. Investigative Ophthalmology and Visual Science 2011;52(9):6081-8.

29. Fu Q, Xu J-W. Effect of intervention via mid-long term follow-up on visual recovery of patients with diabetic retinopathy. Chin J Clin Rehab 2006;10(40):19-21.

30. Gangnon RE, Davis MD, Hubbard LD, et al. A severity scale for diabetic macular edema developed from ETDRS data. Invest Ophthalmol Vis Sci 2008;49(11):5041-7.

31. Gheorghiu M. [The effects of photocoagulation on the electrical activity of the diabetic retina]. [Romanian]. Oftalmologia 2000;51(2):29-34.

32. Gheorghiu M. [Electrical changes in the middle retinal layer in diabetic retinopathy]. [Romanian]. Oftalmologia 2001;53(3):61-5.

33. Gheorghiu M. [Electrical changes in the external retinal layer in the course of diabetic retinopathy (Electroretinographic study)]. [Romanian]. Oftalmologia 2001;52(2):58-62.

34. Gilmore ED, Hudson C, Nrusimhadevara RK, et al. Retinal arteriolar hemodynamic response to an acute hyperglycemic provocation in early and sight-threatening diabetic retinopathy. Microvas Res 2007;73(3):191-7.

35. Gonzalez Villalpando ME, Gonzalez VC, Arredondo PB, et al. Moderate-to-severe diabetic retinopathy is more prevalent in Mexico City than in San Antonio, Texas. Diabetes Care 1997;20(5):773-7.

36. Guleria S, Aggarwal S, Bansal VK, et al. The first successful simultaneous pancreas-kidney transplant in India. Natl Med J India 2005;18(1):18-9.

37. Gupta SK, Viswanath K, Thulasiraj RD, et al. The development of the Indian vision function questionnaire: field testing and psychometric evaluation. Br J Ophthalmol 2005;89(5):621-7.

38. Hanninen J, Takala J, Keinanen-Kiukaanniemi S. Quality of life in NIDDM patients assessed with the SF-20 questionnaire. Diabetes Res Clin Pract 1998;42(1):17-27.

39. Hariprasad SM, Mieler WF, Grassi M, et al. Vision-related quality of life in patients with diabetic macular oedema. Br J Ophthalmol 2008;92(1):89-92.

40. Haritoglou C, Gerss J, Sauerland C, et al. Effect of calcium dobesilate on occurrence of diabetic macular oedema (CALDIRET study): randomised, double-blind, placebo-controlled, multicentre trial. Lancet 2009;373(9672):1364-71.

41. Hawkins WR. Diabetic retinopathy and sodium intake. Arch Ophthalmol 2010;128(8):1085.

42. Henricsson M, Nystrom L, Blohme G, et al. The incidence of retinopathy 10 years after diagnosis in young adult people with diabetes: results from the nationwide population-based Diabetes Incidence Study in Sweden (DISS). Diabetes Care 2003;26(2):349-54.

43. Hirowatari T. Evaluation of a new preoperative ophthalmic solution. Can J Ophthalmol 2005;(1):58-62.

44. Huang ES, Brown SE, Ewigman BG, et al. Patient perceptions of quality of life with diabetes-related complications and treatments. Diabetes Care 2007;30(10):2478-83.

45. Jahn CE, Topfner von SK, Richter J, et al. Improvement of visual acuity in eyes with diabetic macular edema after treatment with pars plana vitrectomy. Ophthalmologica 2004;218(6):378-84.

46. Joussen AM, Weiss C, Bauer D, et al. Triamcinolone versus inner-limiting membrane peeling in persistent diabetic macular edema (TIME study): design issues and implications. Graefes Arch Clin Exp Ophthalmol 2007;245(12):1781-7.

47. Karel I, Kalvodova B. Long-term results of pars plana vitrectomy and silicone oil for complications of diabetic retinopathy. Eur J Ophthalmol 1994;4(1):52-8.

48. Kawashima D, Ohno T, Kinoshita O, et al. Prevalence of vitreous hemorrhage following coronary revascularization in patients with diabetic retinopathy. Cir J 2011;75(2):329-35.

49. Kean-Cowdin R, Varma R, Hays RD, et al. Longitudinal changes in visual acuity and health-related quality of life: the Los Angeles Latino Eye study. Ophthalmology 1907;117(10):1900-7.

50. Keeffe JE, Lam D, Cheung A, et al. Impact of vision impairment on functioning. Aust N Z J Ophthalmol 1998;26:Suppl-8.

51. Klein R, Moss SE, Klein BE, et al. The NEI-VFQ-25 in people with long-term type 1 diabetes mellitus: the Wisconsin Epidemiologic Study of Diabetic Retinopathy. Arch Ophthalmol 2001;119(5):733-40.

52. Knudtson MD, Klein BE, Klein R, et al. Age-related eye disease, quality of life, and functional activity. Arch Ophthalmol 2005;123(6):807-14.

53. Korkeliia MT, Tsupkiridze LR, Kurashvili RB, et al. Psychopathologic peculiarities in patients with diabetes mellitus and non-proliferative retinopathy. Georgian Med News 2009;(166):54-7.

54. Lamoureux EL, Hassell JB, Keeffe JE. The impact of diabetic retinopathy on participation in daily living. Arch Ophthalmol 2004;122(1):84-8.

55. Lee SJ, Sicari C, Harper CA, et al. Examination compliance and screening for diabetic retinopathy: a 2-year follow-up study. Clin Experiment Ophthalmol 2000;28(3):149-52.

56. Leksell JK, Johansson I, Wibell LB, et al. Power and self-perceived health in blind diabetic and nondiabetic individuals. J Adv Nurs 2001;34(4):511-9.

57. Leksell JK, Wikblad KF, Sandberg GE. Sense of coherence and power among people with blindness caused by diabetes. Diabetes Res Clin Pract 2005;67(2):124-9.

58. Leksell JK, Sandberg GE, Wikblad KF. Self-perceived health and self-care among diabetic subjects with defective vision: a comparison between subjects with threat of blindness and blind subjects. J Diabet Complications 2005;19(1):54-9.

59. Lloyd CE, Orchard TJ. Physical and psychological well-being in adults with Type 1 diabetes. Diabetes Res Clin Pract 1999;44(1):9-19.

60. Luckie R, Leese G, McAlpine R, et al. Fear of visual loss in patients with diabetes: Results of the Prevalence of Diabetic Eye Disease in Tayside, Scotland (P-DETS) study. Diabet Med 2007;24(10):1086-92.

61. Maia OO, Jr., Takahashi WY, Bonanomi MT, et al. Visual stability in diabetic retinopathy treated by panretinal laser photocoagulation. Arq Bras Endocrinol Metabol 2007;51(4):575-80.

62. Maia OO, Jr., Takahashi WY, Sampaio MW, et al. Contrast sensitivity in diabetic retinopathy treated with argon laser panphotocoagulation. Arq Bras Oftalmol 2007;70(5):763-6.

63. Mason JO, III, Yunker JJ, Vail R, et al. Intravitreal bevacizumab (Avastin) prevention of panretinal photocoagulation-induced complications in patients with severe proliferative diabetic retinopathy. Retina 2008;28(9):1319-24.

64. Mata Cases M, Roset Gamisans M, Badia Llach X, et al. Effect of type-2 diabetes mellitus on the quality of life of patients treated at primary care consultations in Spain. Aten Prim 2003;31(8):493-9.

65. Mazhar K, Varma R, Choudhury F, et al. Severity of Diabetic Retinopathy and Health-Related Quality of Life The Los Angeles Latino Eye Study. Ophthalmology 2011;118(4):649-55.

66. Murthy GV, Gupta SK, Thulasiraj RD, et al. The development of the Indian vision function questionnaire: questionnaire content. Br J Ophthalmol 2005;89(4):498-503.

67. Nawrocki J, Chrzanowski W, Koch D, et al. Vitreoretinal surgery in diabetic patients on hemodialysis. Eur J Ophthalmol 1997;7(3):283-7.

68. Nemeth B, Hudomel J, Farkas A. Effect of calcium dobesilate (Doxium) on circulatory disorders of the retina with special emphasis on diabetic retinopathy. Ophthalmologica 1975;170(5):434-45.

69. Ramalho LH, Avila MP, Moraes Junior HV, et al. Subclinical diabetic macular edema and mild non-proliferative diabetic retinopathy: data correlation with the retinal thickness analyzer (RTA). Arq Bras Oftalmol 2009;72(4):503-8.

70. Ramezani AR, Ahmadieh H, Ghaseminejad AK, et al. Effect of tranexamic acid on early postvitrectomy diabetic haemorrhage; a randomised clinical trial. Br J Ophthalmol 2005;89(8):1041-4.

71. Real FJ, Brown GC, Brown HC, et al. The effect of comorbidities upon ocular and systemic health-related quality of life. Br J Ophthalmol 2008;92(6):770-4.

72. Robertson N, Burden ML, Burden AC. Psychological morbidity and problems of daily living in people with visual loss and diabetes: do they differ from people without diabetes? Diabet Med 2006;23(10):1110-6.

73. Rohrschneider K, Bruder I, Aust R, et al. Use of a new optoelectronic vision aid for highly visually handicapped patients. Klin Monatsbl Augenheilkd 1997;210(2):105-10.

74. Rossi GC, Milano G, Tinelli C. The Italian version of the 25-item National Eye Institute Visual Function Questionnaire: translation, validity, and reliability. J Glaucoma 2003;12(3):213-20.

75. Roy A, Roy M. Depressive symptoms in African-American type 1 diabetics. Depress Anxiety 2001;13(1):28-31.

76. Sakamaki H, Ikeda S, Ikegami N, et al. Measurement of HRQL using EQ-5D in patients with type 2 diabetes mellitus in Japan. Value Health 2006;9(1):47-53.

77. Sasaki S, Tsuru NE, Inoguchi T, et al. Incidence of latent depression associated with diabetic retinopathy and utility of SRQ-D in diagnosis. [Japanese]. Folia Ophthalmol Jpn 2005;56(6):401-5.

78. Scalinci SZ, Simoni P, Scorolli L, et al. Visual rehabilitation in advanced diabetic retinopathy. Ann Ottalmol Clin Ocul 1997;123(3):161-8.

79. Schweitzer KD, Eneh AA, Hurst J, et al. Visual function analysis in acute posterior vitreous detachment. Can J Ophthalmol 2011;46(3):232-6.

80. Searle A, Wetherell MA, Campbell R, et al. Do patients' beliefs about type 2 diabetes differ in accordance with complications: an investigation into diabetic foot ulceration and retinopathy. Int J Behav Med 2008;15(3):173-9.

81. Sharma S, Brown GC, Brown MM, et al. The cost-effectiveness of grid laser photocoagulation for the treatment of diabetic macular edema: results of a patient-based cost-utility analysis. Curr Opin Ophthalmol 2000;11(3):175-9.

82. Sharma S, Hollands H, Brown GC, et al. The cost-effectiveness of early vitrectomy for the treatment of vitreous hemorrhage in diabetic retinopathy. Curr Opin Ophthalmol 2001;12(3):230-4.

83. Sharma S, Oliver-Fernandez A, Bakal J, et al. Utilities associated with diabetic retinopathy: results from a Canadian sample. Br J Ophthalmol 2003;87(3):259-61.

84. Shimura M, Yasuda K, Shiono T. Posterior sub-Tenon's capsule injection of triamcinolone acetonide prevents panretinal photocoagulation-induced visual dysfunction in patients with severe diabetic retinopathy and good vision. Ophthalmology 2006;113(3):381-7.

85. Sjolie AK, Klein R, Porta M, et al. Effect of candesartan on progression and regression of retinopathy in type 2 diabetes (DIRECT-Protect 2): a randomised placebo-controlled trial. Lancet 2008;372(9647):1385-93.

86. Smith DH, Johnson ES, Russell A, et al. Lower visual acuity predicts worse utility values among patients with type 2 diabetes. Qual Life Res 2008;17(10):1277-84.

87. Smith TS, Szetu J, Bourne RR. The prevalence and severity of diabetic retinopathy, associated risk factors and vision loss in patients registered with type 2 diabetes in Luganville, Vanuatu. Br J Ophthalmol 2007;91(4):415-9.

88. Sugitani A, Hotta K, Suzuki T, et al. Daily activities of patients with low vision associated with diabetic ocular complications. Folia Ophthalmol Jpn 2003;54(12):952-5.

89. Takeda M. Validity of low-vision aids for patients with vision impairment due to diabetic retinopathy. Folia Ophthalmol Jpn 2003;54(12):947-51.

90. Trento M, Tomelini M, Lattanzio R, et al. Perception of, and anxiety levels induced by, laser treatment in patients with sight-threatening diabetic retinopathy. A multicentre study. Diabet Med 2006;23(10):1106-9.

91. van Nispen RM, de Boer MR, Hoeijmakers JG, et al. Co-morbidity and visual acuity are risk factors for health-related quality of life decline: five-month follow-up EQ-5D data of visually impaired older patients. Health Qual Life Ooutcomes 2009;7:18.

92. Verma SK, Luo N, Subramaniam M, et al. Impact of depression on health related quality of life in patients with diabetes. Ann Acad Med Singap 2010;39(12):913-9.

93. Williams GP, Pathak-Ray V, Austin MW, et al. Quality of life and visual rehabilitation: an observational study of low vision in three general practices in West Glamorgan. Eye 2007;21(4):522-7.

94. Wu WC, Hsu KH, Chen TL, et al. Interventions for relieving pain associated with panretinal photocoagulation: a prospective randomized trial. Eye 2006;20(6):712-9.

95. Yalcin BM, Karahan TF, Ozcelik M, et al. The effects of an emotional intelligence program on the quality of life and well-being of patients with type 2 diabetes mellitus. Diabetes Educ 2008;34(6):1013-24.

96. Yamada Y, Hirasawa Y, Ohishi M, et al. Rehabilitation of the once-sighted blind report 8 - employment of visually impaired and blind. Folia Ophthalmol Jpn 2003;54(1):16-20.

97. Yamada Y, Hirasawa Y, Takasawa T, et al. Vision rehabilitation for the once-sighted blind report 9 - frequency and characteristics of sleep disturbance and depression among visually impaired patients. Folia Ophthalmol Jpn 2004;55(3):192-6.

98. Yamada Y, Hirasawa Y, Ohishi M, et al. Improving independence of the visually impaired - effectiveness of a vision clinic and personal computer class. Folia Ophthalmol Jpn 2004;55(4):265-9.

99. Yeoh J, Williams C, Allen P, et al. Avastin as an adjunct to vitrectomy in the management of severe proliferative diabetic retinopathy: a prospective case series. Clin Experiment Ophthalmol 2008;36(5):449-54.

Outcome (n = 185)

1. Effect of 6 months of strict metabolic control on eye and kidney function in insulin-dependent diabetics with background retinopathy. Steno study group. Lancet 1982 Jan;(8264):121-4.

2. The effect of intensive diabetes therapy on the development and progression of neuropathy. The Diabetes Control and Complications Trial Research Group. Ann Intern Med 1995 Apr 15;122(8):561-8.

3. Even modest improvements in blood sugar control can substantially improve quality of life for people with diabetes. AHRQ Research Activities 1998 Nov;(221):2.

4. Retinopathy and nephropathy in patients with type 1 diabetes four years after a trial of intensive therapy. The Diabetes Control and Complications Trial/Epidemiology of Diabetes Interventions and Complications Research Group. New Engl J Med 2000 Feb 10;342(6):381-9.

5. Abdoli S, Ashktorab T, Ahmadi F, Parvizi S, et al. The empowerment process in people with diabetes: an Iranian perspective. Int Nurs Rev 2008 Dec;55(4):447-53.

6. Ahmadian L, Moradi II, Lopez JA, Mayers .M., et al. Diabetes Conference: 69th Annual Meeting of the American Diabetes Association New Orleans, LA United 2009.

7. Ahola AJ, Saraheimo M, Forsblom C, Hietala K, et al. Health-related quality of life in patients with type 1 diabetes-association with diabetic complications (the FinnDiane Study). Nephrol Dial Transplant 2010 Jun;25(6):1903-8.

8. Airaksinen KE, Salmela PI, Miettinen RU, Ikaheimo MJ, et al. Effect of coronary artery bypass surgery on autonomic nervous function and retinopathy in diabetic patients. Diabetes Res 1990 Jul;14(3):149-50.

9. Akatsuka R. [Quantification of anxiety of patients by their expression and complaints--innovation in nursing of patients with vision disorders caused by diabetes mellitus]. [Japanese]. Kango Gijutsu 1987 Feb;33(3):268-72.

10. Al-Ansari SA, Tennant MTS, Greve MDJ, Hinz BJ, et al. Short report: suboptimal diabetes care in high-risk diabetic patients attending a specialist retina clinic. Diabet Med 2009 Dec;26(12):1296-300.

11. Al-Ghamdi AA. A high prevalence of depression among diabetic patients at a teaching hospital in Western Saudi Arabia. Neurosciences 2004 Apr;9(2):108-12.

12. Al-Tuwijri AA, Al-Doghether MH, Akturk Z, Al-Megbil TI. Quality of life of people with diabetes attending primary care health centres in Riyadh: bad control -- good quality? Quality in Primary Care 2007 Oct;15(5):307-14.

13. Almond C, Hayward E, Freemantle N, Brereton NJ. The use of a mixed-treatment comparison to assess the costeffectiveness of ozurdex (dexamethasone intravitreal implant in applicator) compared with bevacizumab intravitreal injections for patients with macular oedema following branch retinal vein occlusion. 5-8 November 2011, Madrid, Spain 2011.

14. Amsberg S, Anderbro T, Wredling R, Lisspers J, et al. A cognitive behavior therapy-based intervention among poorly controlled adult type 1 diabetes patients-A randomized controlled trial. Patient Educ Couns 2009;77(1):72-80.

15. Anaforoglu I, Atasoy V, Algn E, Kutanis R. Endocrine Abstracts Conference: 12th European Congress of Endocrinology 2010; 272.

16. Ando N, Iwaki H. An attempt to better control diabetic retinopathy. [Japanese]. Folia Ophthal Jap 2000;51(3):287-290.

17. Araki A, Izumo Y, Inoue J, Takahashi R, et al. Factors associated with increased diabetes burden in elderly diabetic patients. Nippon Ronen Igakkai Zasshi 1995 Dec;32(12):797-803.

18. Arevalo JF, Sanchez JG, Fromow-Guerra J, Wu L, et al. Comparison of two doses of primary intravitreal bevacizumab (Avastin) for diffuse diabetic macular edema: results from the Pan-American Collaborative Retina Study Group (PACORES) at 12-month follow-up. Graefes Archive for Clin Exp Ophthalmol 2009 Jun;247(6):735-43.

19. Bagust A, Beale S. Modelling EuroQol health-related utility values for diabetic complications from CODE-2 data. Health Econ 2005 Mar;14(3):217-30.

20. Bailey CC, Sparrow JM. Visual symptomatology in patients with sight-threatening diabetic retinopathy. Diabet Med 2001;18(11):883-8.

21. Baker RS, Bazargan M, Calderon JL, Hays RD. Psychometric Performance of the National Eye Institute Visual Function Questionnaire in Latinos and Non-Latinos. Ophthalmology 2006;113(8).

22. Balarin S, V, Temporini ER, De Carvalho Moreira FD, Kara-Jose N. Treatment of diabetic retinopathy: Patients' perceptions in Rio Claro (Sao Paulo State) - Brazil. Arq Bras Oftalmol 2005 May;68(3):363-8.

23. Bek T, Moller F, Klausen B. Short item visual prognosis after retinal laser photocoagulation for diabetic maculopathy. Acta Ophthalmol Scand 2000;78(5):539-42.

24. Bernbaum M, Albert SG, Brusca SR, Drimmer A, et al. A model clinical program for patients with diabetes and vision impairment. Diabetes Educ 1989 Jul;15(4):325-30.

25. Bickerdike C, Mellor CM. ROP rivisited: a survey of adults with residual vision... retinopathy of prematurity. J Vis Impair Blind 2001 Dec;95(12):749-51.

26. Brands AMA, Van Den Berg E, Manschot SM, Biessels GJ, et al. A detailed profile of cognitive dysfunction and its relation to psychological distress in patients with type 2 diabetes mellitus. J Int Neuropsychol Soc 2007;13(2):288-97.

27. Brennig C, Schollbauer V, Walter E, Gallagher M, et al. Economic evaluation of ranibizumab in the treatment of visual impairment due to diabetic macular edema in Austria. 5-8 November 2011, Madrid Spain 2011 p. A478.

28. Brose LS, Bradley C. Psychometric development of the retinopathy treatment satisfaction questionnaire (RetTSQ). Psychol Health Med 2009 Dec;14(6):740-54.

29. Brose LS, Bradley C. Psychometric development of the individualized Retinopathy-Dependent Quality of Life questionnaire (RetDQoL). Value Health 2010 Jan;13(1):119-27.

30. Brown DM, Campochiaro PA, Bhisitkul RB, et al. Sustained benefits from ranibizumab for macular edema following branch retinal vein occlusion: 12-month outcomes of a phase III study. Ophthalmology 2011;118(8):1594-602.

31. Brown GC, Brown MM, Sharma S, Brown H, et al. Quality of life associated with diabetes mellitus in an adult population. J Diabetes Complications 2000 Jan;14(1):18-24.

32. Brown MM, Brown GC, Sharma S, Busbee B, et al. Quality of life associated with visual loss. Evid Based Eye Care 2003 Oct;4(4):212-3.

33. Brown SES, Meltzer DO, Chin MH, Huang ES. Perceptions of quality-of-life effects of treatments for diabetes mellitus in vulnerable and nonvulnerable older patients. J Am Geriatr Soc 2008 Jul;56(7):1183-90.

34. Bursell SE, Clermont AC, Aiello LP, Schlossman DK, et al. High-dose vitamin E supplementation normalizes retinal blood flow and creatinine clearance in patients with type 1 diabetes. Diabetes Care 1999 Aug;(8):1245-51.

35. Burton AJ, Reynolds A, O'Neill D. Sildenafil (Viagra) a cause of proliferative diabetic retinopathy? Eye 2000 Oct;14(Pt 5):785-6.

36. Chang K. Comorbidities, quality of life and patients' willingness to pay for a cure for type 2 diabetes in Taiwan. Public Health 2010 May;124(5):284-94.

37. Chang P-Y, Yang C-M, Yang C-H, Chen M-S, et al. Pars plana vitrectomy for diabetic fibrovascular proliferation with and without internal limiting membrane peeling. Eye 2009 Apr;23(4):960-5.

38. Chatziralli IP, Kanonidou E, Papazisis L. Frequency of fundus pathology related to patients' dissatisfaction after phacoemulsification cataract surgery. Bulletin de la Societe Belge d Ophtalmologie 2011;(317):21-4.

39. Chen P, He X-G. Visual function of patients with diabetic retinopathy and the intervention of dan-shen root: Quantified evaluation of sight and visual acuity. Chin J Clin Rehab 2005 Jun 21;9(23):124-6.

40. Chuang L-M, Tsai ST, Huang BY, Tai TY. The status of diabetes control in Asia - A cross-sectional survey of 24 317 patients with diabetes mellitus in 1998. Diabet Med 2002;19(12):978-85.

41. Chui L. Fifteen Year Followup of the Ocular and Medical Status of Early Treatment Diabetic Retinopathy Study (ETDRS) Patients Enrolled at the Joslin Diabetes Center. IOVS 2005;ARVO-abstract.

42. Cruickshanks KJ, Moss SE, Klein R, Klein BE. Physical activity and the risk of progression of retinopathy or the development of proliferative retinopathy. Ophthalmology 1995 Aug;102(8):1177-82.

43. Cugati S, Kifley A, Mitchell P, Wang JJ. Temporal trends in the age-specific prevalence of diabetes and diabetic retinopathy in older persons: Population-based survey findings. Diabetes Res Clin Pract 2006 Dec;74(3):301-8.

44. Cumba RJ, Al-Attar L. Clinical and Translational Science Conference: 2010 Clinical and Translational Research and Education Meeting: ACRT 2010;S24.

45. De Mendonca RHF, Zihlmann KF, Freire ML, De Salles Oliveira RC, et al. Quality of life in patients with Proliferative Diabetic Retinopathy. Rev Bras Oftalmol 2008;67(4):177-83.

46. De Visser CL, Bilo HJG, Groenier KH, De Visser W, et al. The influence of cardiovascular disease on quality of life in type 2 diabetics. Qual Life Res 2002;11(3):249-61.

47. Didjurgeit U, Kruse J, Schmitz N, Stuckenschneider P, et al. A time-limited, problem-orientated psychotherapeutic intervention in Type 1 diabetic patients with complications: a randomized controlled trial. Diabet Med 2002 Oct;19(10):814-21.

48. Donnio-Cordoba A, Richer R, Spinelli F, Merle H. Diabetic retinopathy in Martinique: results of a cross-sectional survey based on 771 patients. Journal Francais d Opthalmologie 2001 Jun;24(6):603-9.

49. Dreer LE, Elliott TR, Fletcher DC, Swanson M. Social problem-solving abilities and psychological adjustment of persons in low vision rehabilitation. Rehabil Psychol 2005;50(3):232-8.

50. El-Asrar AM, Al-Rubeaan KA, Al-Amro SA, Kangave D, et al. Risk factors for diabetic retinopathy among Saudi diabetics. Int Ophthalmol 1998;22(3):155-61.

51. Escarce JJ, Kapur K, Solomon MD, Mangione CM, et al. Practice characteristics and HMO enrollee satisfaction with specialty care: an analysis of patients with glaucoma and diabetic retinopathy. Health Serv Res 2003 Aug;38(4):1135-55.

52. Fevzi A, Aysegul Y. Psychometric performance of the National Eye Institute 25-Item Visual Function Questionnaire: In Turkish diabetic retinopathy patients. The Patient: Patient-Centered Outcomes Research 2008;1(2):115-25.

53. Fonda SJ, Bursell SE, Lewis DG, Garren J, et al. The relationship of a diabetes telehealth eye care program to standard eye care and change in diabetes health outcomes. Telemed J E Health 2007 Dec;13(6):635-44.

54. Fraenkel G, Comaish I, Lawless MA, Kelly MR, et al. Development of a Questionnaire to Assess Subjective Vision Score in Myopes Seeking Refractive Surgery. J Refractive Surg 2004;20(1):10-9.

55. Fukino O, Shinzato R, Ishizu H, Tamai H. Psychological features of diabetics with severe complications (retinopathy). J Jpn Diabetes Soc 1985;28(8):889-94.

56. Gabrielian A, Hariprasad SM, Jager RD, Green JL, et al. The utility of visual function questionnaire in the assessment of the impact of diabetic retinopathy on vision-related quality of life. Eye 2010 Jan;24(1):29-35.

57. Gardner TW, Miller ML, Cunningham D, Blankenship GW. The retinal depression sign in diabetic retinopathy. Graefes Archive for Clin Exp Ophthalmol 1995 Oct;233(10):617-20.

58. Gendelman N, Snell-Bergeon JK, McFann K, Kinney G, et al. Prevalence and correlates of depression in individuals with and without type 1 diabetes. Diabetes Care 2009 Apr;32(4):575-9.

59. Goddijn P, Bilo H, Meadows K, Groenier K, et al. The validity and reliability of the Diabetes Health Profile (DHP) in NIDDM patients referred for insulin therapy. Qual Life Res 1996 Aug;5(4):433-42.

60. Gottsater A, Kangro M, Sundkvist G. Early parasympathetic neuropathy associated with elevated fasting plasma C-peptide concentrations and late parasympathetic neuropathy with hyperglycaemia and other microvascular complications. Diabet Med 2004 Dec;21(12):1304-9.

61. Graham JE, Stoebner-May DG, Ostir GV, Al Snih S, et al. Health related quality of life in older Mexican Americans with diabetes: A cross-sectional study. Health Qual Life Outcomes 2007;5.

62. Haber LD. Disabling effects of chronic disease and impairment. J Chronic Dis 1971 Sep;24(7):469-87.

63. Hahl J, Hamalainen H, Sintonen H, Simell T, et al. Health-related quality of life in type 1 diabetes without or with symptoms of long-term complications. Qual Life Res 2002;11(5):427-36.

64. Hahl J, Hamalainen H, Simell T, Simell O. The effects of type 1 diabetes and its long-term complications on physical and mental health status. Pharmacoeconomics 2006;24(6):559-69.

65. Haig J, Lawrence D, Barbeau M, Blouin J, et al. Economic evaluation of ranibizumab for the treatment of diabetic macular edema in Canada.: May 2011, Baltimore, MD; 2011 p. A96-7.

66. Hanninen J, Keinanen-Kiukaanniemi S, Takala J. Population-based audit of non-insulin-dependent diabetic patients aged under 65 years in primary health care. Scand J Prim Health Care 1998 Dec;16(4):227-32.

67. Harris EL, Sherman SH, Georgopoulos A. Black-white differences in risk of developing retinopathy among individuals with type 2 diabetes. Diabetes Care 1999 May;22(5):779-83.

68. Hart HE, Bilo HJG, Redekop WK, Stolk RP, et al. Quality of life of patients with type I diabetes mellitus. Qual Life Res 2003 Dec;12(8):1089-97.

69. Hart HE, Redekop WK, Bilo HJG, Meyboom-de JB, et al. Health related quality of life in patients with type I diabetes mellitus: Generic & disease-specific measurement. Indian J Med Res 2007 Mar;125(3):203-16.

70. Harzallah F, Alberti H, Kanoun F, Elhouch F, et al. Quality of care of patients with type 2 diabetes in a Tunisian university hospital. Diabetes Metab 2004 Dec;30(6):523-6.

71. Hayashi K, Igarashi C, Hirata A, Hayashi H. Changes in diabetic macular oedema after phacoemulsification surgery. Eye 2009 Feb;23(2):389-96.

72. Hayward E, Almond C, Trueman D, Yeh WS, et al. The cost-effectiveness of ozurdex (dexamethasone intravitreal implant in applicator) compared with observation for the treatment of macular oedema following central and branch retinal vein occlusion. 5-8 November 2011, Madrid, Spain 2011 p. A506.

73. Heggie J. Effectiveness of diabetes eye health education during retinal screening. Diabetes Prim Care 2002 May;4(3):90-5.

74. Heller S, Evans AT, Kazlauskaite R. Training in flexible intensive insulin management improved glycaemic control and quality of life in type 1 diabetes. Evid Based Med 2003 May;8(3):80.

75. Henricsson M, Heijl A. The effect of panretinal laser photocoagulation on visual acuity, visual fields and on subjective visual impairment in preproliferative and early proliferative diabetic retinopathy. Acta Ophthalmol 1994 Oct;72(5):570-5.

76. Herpertz S, Johann B, Lichtblau K, Stadtb+ñumer M, et al. Psychosocial stress and use of psychosocial support in patients with diabetes mellitus. Med Klin 2000;95(7):369-77.

77. Hollands H, Lam M, Pater J, Sharma S, et al. Reliability of the time trade-off technique of utility assessment in patients with retinal disease. Evid Based Eye Care 2002 Jul;3(3):168-9.

78. Hoogma RPLM, Spijker AJM, van Doorn-Scheele M, van Doorn TT, et al. Quality of life and metabolic control in patients with diabetes mellitus type I treated by continuous subcutaneous insulin infusion or multiple daily insulin injections. Neth J Med 2004 Nov;62(10):383-7.

79. Huang IC, Liu JH, Wu AW, Wu MY, et al. Evaluating the reliability, validity and minimally important difference of the Taiwanese version of the diabetes quality of life (DQOL) measurement. Health Qual Life Outcomes 2008;6:87.

80. Huang IC, Hwang CC, Wu MY, Lin W, et al. Diabetes-specific or generic measures for health-related quality of life? Evidence from psychometric validation of the D-39 and SF–36. Value Health 2008 May;11(3):450-61.

81. Inoda S, Shimizu Y, Makino S. Vitrectomy for proliferative diabetic retinopathy. [Japanese]. Folia Ophthal Jap 1996; 47(4):460-4.

82. Ishii H. Psychosocial problems and their management in patients with diabetic retinopathy. [Japanese]. Folia Ophthal Jap 1996;47(1):22-7.

83. Iyigun E, Bayer A, Tastan S, Demiralp M, et al. Validity and reliability study for the NEI-VFO-39 scale in chronic ophthalmic diseases - Turkish version. Acta Ophthalmol 2010 Jun;88(4):e115-e119.

84. Jacko JA, Barnard L, Yi JS, Edwards PJ, et al. Empirical validation of the WINDOWS accessibility settings and multimodal feedback for a menu selection task for users with diabetic retinopathy. Behav Info Tech 2005 Nov;24(6):419-34.

85. Jacobson AM, Rand LI, Hauser ST. Psychologic stress and glycemic control: a comparison of patients with and without proliferative diabetic retinopathy. Psychosom Med 1985 Jul;47(4):372-81.

86. Jones HL, Walker EA, Schechter CB, Blanco E. Vision is precious: a successful behavioral intervention to increase the rate of screening for diabetic retinopathy for inner-city adults. Diabetes Educ 2010 Jan;36(1):118-26.

87. Joussen AM. Triamcinolone versus Inner-Limiting Membrane Peeling for Diffuse Macular Edema (TIME Study): Design Issues and Implications. IOVS 2005;Vol-abstract.

88. Kamel HK, Shareeff M, Guro-Razuman S, Mir T. Vision impairment and impact on functional and psychological assessments in elderly patients. J Invest Med 1999;47(2).

89. Karel I, Kalvodova B, Kondrova J, Bedrich P, et al. [Is the prognosis of pars plana vitrectomy in diabetic retinopathy dependent on the general status of the diabetic?]. [Czech]. Ceskoslovenska Oftalmologie 1989 Mar;45(2):77-83.

90. Karlson B, Agardh CD. Burden of illness, metabolic control, and complications in relation to depressive symptoms in IDDM patients. Diabet Med 1997 Dec;14(12):1066-72.

91. Kawashima D, Ohno T, Kinoshita O, et al. Prevalence of vitreous hemorrhage following coronary revascularization in patients with diabetic retinopathy. Circulation Journal 2011;75(2):329-35.

92. Kempen JH, O'Colmain BJ, Leske MC, Haffner SM, et al. The prevalence of diabetic retinopathy among adults in the United States. Arch Ophthalmol 2004 Apr;122(4):552-63.

93. Khatib FA, Jarrah NS, Shegem NS, Bateiha AM, et al. Sexual dysfunction among Jordanian men with diabetes. Saudi Medical Journal 2006 Mar;27(3):351-6.

94. Kinder LS, Katon WJ, Ludman E, Russo J, et al. Improving depression care in patients with diabetes and multiple complications. J Gen Intern Med 2006;21(10):1036-41.

95. Klein R, Klein BE, Moss SE, Cruickshanks KJ. The Wisconsin Epidemiologic Study of Diabetic Retinopathy: XVII. The 14-year incidence and progression of diabetic retinopathy and associated risk factors in type 1 diabetes. Ophthalmology 1998 Oct;105(10):1801-15.

96. Klein R, Moss SE, Klein BEK, Gutierrez P, et al. The NEI-VFQ-25 in people with long-term type 1 diabetes mellitus: The Wisconsin epidemiology study of diabetic retinopathy. Evid Based Eye Care 2002 Jan;3(1):60-1.

97. Knudsen MS, Thomas S, Gallagher M, Mitchell P. Assessment of utility loss from diabetic macular edema based on restore trial. Value in Health 2011; 14(7).

98. Koerner F, Koerner U, Eichenseher N. Diabetic retinopathy study. Data acquisition and its reliability. Albrecht Von Graefes Archiv fur Klinische und Experimentelle Ophthalmologie 1977 May 23;202(3):163-73.

99. Komatsu M, Kifune M, Shimizu Y, Nawashima M. Social support for patients with visual disorders - The role of social workers. Folia Ophthalmol Jpn 1996;47(1):32-6.

100. Koopmanschap M. Coping with Type II diabetes: The patient's perspective. Diabetologia 2002;45(6).

101. Kunimatsu S, Kato S, Sumi I, Kitazawa M, et al. Evaluation of quality of life characteristics and grade of legal visual impairment. Nippon Ganka Gakkai Zasshi 2007 Jun;111(6):454-8.

102. Kwiatkowski A, Michalak G, Czerwinski J, Wszola M, et al. Quality of life after simultaneous pancreas-kidney transplantation. Transplant Proc 2005 Oct;37(8):3558-9.

103. Lamoureux EL, Hassell JB, Keeffe JE. The determinants of participation in activities of daily living in people with impaired vision. Am J Ophthalmol 2004;137(2):265-70.

104. Lamoureux EL, Pallant JF, Pesudovs K, Hassell JB, et al. The impact of vision impairment questionnaire: An evaluation of its measurement properties using Rasch analysis. Invest Ophthalmol Vis Sci 2006;47(11):4732-41.

105. Lamoureux EL, Tee HW, Pesudovs K, Pallant JF, et al. Can clinicians use the PHQ-9 to assess depression in people with vision loss? Optom Vis Sci 2009;86(2):139-45.

106. Lamoureux EL, Pesudovs K, Thumboo J, Saw SM, et al. An evaluation of the reliability and validity of the visual functioning questionnaire (VF-11) using rasch analysis in an Asian population. Invest Ophthalmol Vis Sci 2009;50(6):2607-13.

107. Langelaan M, de Boer MR, van Nispen RM, Wouters B, et al. Impact of visual impairment on quality of life: a comparison with quality of life in the general population and with other chronic conditions. Ophthalmic Epidemiol 2007 May;14(3):119-26.

108. Larsson D, Lager I, Nilsson PM. Socio-economic characteristics and quality of life in diabetes mellitus--relation to metabolic control. Scand J Public Health 1999 Jun;27(2):101-5.

109. Lee HJ, Chapa D, Kao CW, Jones D, et al. Depression, quality of life, and glycemic control in individuals with type 2 diabetes. J Am Acad Nurse Pract 2009 Apr;21(4):214-24.

110. Lin J-C, Chie W-C. Psychometric validation of the Taiwan Chinese version of the 25-Item National Eye Institute Visual Functioning Questionnaire. J Eval Clin Pract 2010 Jun;16(3):619-26.

111. Linder M, Chang TS, Scott IU, Hay D, et al. Validity of the visual function index (VF–14) in patients with retinal disease. Arch Ophthalmol 1999 Dec;117(12):1611-6.

112. Lloyd A, Sawyer W, Hopkinson P. Impact of long-term complications on quality of life in patients with type 2 diabetes not using insulin. Value Health 2001 Sep;4(5):392-400.

113. Lloyd CE, Pambianco G, Orchard TJ. Diabetes Conference: 69th Annual Meeting of the American Diabetes Association New Orleans, LA United States 2009.

114. Lloyd CE, Pambianco G, Orchard TJ. Does diabetes-related distress explain the presence of depressive symptoms and/or poor self-care in individuals with Type 1 diabetes? Diabet Med 2010 Feb;27(2):234-7.

115. Lu Y-W, Ding H-F, Wu X-L, Kong N, et al. Correlative analysis between social support and quality of life in patients with diabetic retinopathy. Chin J Clin Rehab 2005 Feb;9(7):154-5.

116. Lustman PJ, Griffith LS, Clouse RE. Depression in adults with diabetes. Results of 5-yr follow-up study. Diabetes Care 1988 Sep;11(8):605-12.

117. Maddigan SL, Majumdar SR, Toth EL, Feeny DH, et al. Health-related quality of life deficits associated with varying degrees of disease severity in type 2 diabetes. Health Qual Life Outcomes 2003;1.

118. Mangione CM, Berry S, Spritzer K, Janz NK, et al. Identifying the content area for the 51-item National Eye Institute Visual Function Questionnaire: results from focus groups with visually impaired persons. Arch Ophthalmol 1998 Feb;116(2):227-33.

119. Mangione CM, Lee PP, Pitts J, Gutierrez P, et al. Psychometric properties of the National Eye Institute Visual Function Questionnaire (NEI-VFQ). NEI-VFQ Field Test Investigators. Arch Ophthalmol 1998 Nov;116(11):1496-504.

120. Mangione CM, Lee PP, Gutierrez PR, Spritzer K, et al. Development of the 25-item National Eye Institute Visual Function Questionnaire. Arch Ophthalmol 2001 Jul;119(7):1050-8.

121. Mangione CM, Lee PP, Gutierrez PR, Spritzer K, et al. Development of the 25-item National Eye Institute visual function questionnaire. Evid Based Eye Care 2002 Jan;3(1):58-9.

122. Maturi RK, Merrill PT, Lomeo MD, az-Rohena R, et al. Perfluoro-N-octane (PFO) in the repair of complicated retinal detachments due to severe proliferative diabetic retinopathy. Ophthalmic Surg Lasers 1999 Nov;30(9):715-20.

123. McClean MT, Andrews WJ, McElnay JC. Characteristics associated with neuropathy and/or retinopathy in a hospital outpatient diabetic clinic. Pharm World Sci 2005 Jun;27(3):154-8.

124. McCloud C, Harrington A, King L. Understanding people's experience of vitreo-retinal day surgery: A Gadamerian-guided study. J Adv Nurs 2012;68(1):94-103.

125. McNeely MJ, Boyko EJ. Diabetes-related comorbidities in Asian Americans: results of a national health survey. J Diabetes Complications 2005 Mar;19(2):101-6.

126. Miettinen H, Haffner SM, Lehto S, Ronnemaa T, et al. Retinopathy predicts coronary heart disease events in NIDDM patients. Diabetes Care 1996 Dec;19(12):1445-8.

127. Moore JE, Giesen JM, Weber JM, Crews JE. Functional outcomes reported by consumers of the Independent Living Program for Older Individuals Who Are Blind. J Vis Impair Blind 2001 Jul;95(7):403-17.

128. Moore LW, Miller M. Older men's experiences of living with severe visual impairment. J Adv Nurs 2003 Jul;43(1):10-8.

129. Morgan CL, McEwan P, Morrissey M, Peters JR, et al. Characterization and comparison of health-related utility in people with diabetes with various single and multiple vascular complications. Diabet Med 2006 Oct;23(10):1100-5.

130. Moss SE, Klein R, Sjolie AK, et al. Angiotensin receptor blockade not related to history of dry eye symptoms and treatment in The Diabetic Retinopathy Candesartan Trials (DIRECT). Acta Opthalmologica 2011;89(6):e535-e536.

131. Nakatani S, Ishida M, Yanashima K. Problems in low vision patients with diabetic retinopathy. [Japanese]. Folia Ophthal Jap 1997; 48(11):1304-7.

132. Navuluri RB. Diabetic retinopathy screening among Hispanics in Lea County, New Mexico. J Health Care Poor Underserved 2000 Nov;11(4):430-43.

133. Neves C, Carvalheiro M, Ferreira P. Quality of life in people with diabetes mellitus. Arq Med 2002 Jul;16(4-6):200-10.

134. Nguyen TT, Wong TY, Islam FM, Hubbard L, et al. Is depression associated with microvascular disease in patients with type 2 diabetes? Depress Anxiety 2008;25(11):E158-E162.

135. Oehler-Giarratana J, Fitzgerald RG. Group therapy with blind diabetics. Arch Gen Psychiatry 1980 Apr;37(4):463-7.

136. Oehler JW. An exploratory study of psychological reactions to visual loss and blindness in patients with diabetic retinopathy 1984.

137. Pahor D. Visual field loss after argon laser panretinal photocoagulation in diabetic retinopathy: full- versus mild-scatter coagulation. Int Ophthalmol 1998;22(5):313-9.

138. Papadopoulos AA, Kontodimopoulos N, Frydas A, Ikonomakis E, et al. Predictors of health-related quality of life in type II diabetic patients in Greece. BMC Public Health 2007;7.

139. Phillips CJ, Harper GAD, Waheed N, Owens DR, et al. Screening for diabetic retinopathy: The costs to patients - A pilot study. Pract Diabetes Int 1997;14(5):128-31.

140. Quandt SA, Graham CN, Bell RA, Snively BM, et al. Ethnic disparities in health-related quality of life among older rural adults with diabetes. Ethn Dis 2007;17(3):471-6.

141. Ragnarson TG, Apelqvist J. Health-related quality of life in patients with diabetes mellitus and foot ulcers. J Diabetes Complications 2000 Sep;14(5):235-41.

142. Roy MS, Klein R, O'Colmain BJ, Klein BE, et al. The prevalence of diabetic retinopathy among adult type 1 diabetic persons in the United States. Arch Ophthalmol 2004 Apr;122(4):546-51.

143. Roy MS, Roy A, Affouf M. Depression is a risk factor for poor glycemic control and retinopathy in African-Americans with type 1 diabetes. Psychosom Med 2007 Jul;69(6):537-42.

144. Roy MS, Peng B, Roy A. Risk factors for coronary disease and stroke in previously hospitalized African-Americans with Type 1 diabetes: a 6-year follow-up. Diabet Med 2007 Dec;24(12):1361-8.

145. Rubin RJ, Dietrich KA, Hawk AD. Clinical and economic impact of implementing a comprehensive diabetes management program in managed care. J Clin Endocrinol Met 1998;83(8):2635-42.

146. Saatcioglu O, Celikel FC, Kutluturk F, Elbozan Cumurcu B, et al. Disability and quality of life in patients with type 2 diabetes mellitus. Anatolian J Clin Invest 2008;2(3):106-12.

147. Saglam ZA, Saler T, Ataoglu E, Temiz LU, et al. The frequency of depression in turkish patients with diabetes and diabetic complications. Endocrinologist 2010 Jan;20(1):19-22.

148. Sakthong P, Charoenvisuthiwongs R, Shabunthom R. A comparison of EQ-5D index scores using the UK, US, and Japan preference weights in a Thai sample with type 2 diabetes. Health Qual Life Outcomes 2008;6:71.

149. Savli H, Sevinc A. The evaluation of the Turkish version of the Well-being Questionnaire (WBQ-22) in patients with Type 2 diabetes: The effects of diabetic complications. J Endocrinol Invest 2005;28(8):683-91.

150. Scott IU, Smiddy WE, Schiffman J, Feuer WJ, et al. Quality of life of low-vision patients and the impact of low-vision services. Am J Ophthalmol 1999;128(1):54-62.

151. Shah SM, Nguyen QD, Sy JP, Ianchulev. The RIDE and RISE Studies of the Efficacy and Safety of Intravitreal Ranibizumab (LUCENTISA(R)) in Clinically Significant Macular Edema With Center Involvement Secondary to Diabetes Mellitus. IOVS 2011;ARVO-abstract.

152. Shah VA, Gupta SK, Shah KV, Vinjamaram S, et al. TTO utility scores measure quality of life in patients with visual morbidity due to diabetic retinopathy or ARMD. Ophthalmic Epidemiol 2004 Feb;11(1):43-51.

153. Sharma S, Oliver-Fernandez A, Bakal J, Hollands H, et al. Utilities associated with diabetic retinopathy: Results from a Canadian sample. Evid Based Eye Care 2003 Jul;4(3):172-3.

154. Sibay TM, Elder JR, Hausler HR. Incidence of diabetic retinopathy among the mentally ill. Can J Ophthalmol 1971 Jan;6(1):42-5.

155. Slawson D. How often should patients with type 2 diabetes mellitus be screened for retinopathy? Evid Based Pract 2000 May;3(5):2-3.

156. Smith AF. The economic impact of ophthalmic services for persons with diabetes in the Canadian Province of Nova Scotia: 1993-1996. Ophthalmic Epidemiol 2001 Feb;8(1):13-25.

157. Sullivan LM, Dukes KA, Harris L, Dittus RS, et al. A comparison of various methods of collecting self-reported health outcomes data among low-income and minority patients. Med Care 1995 Apr;33(4:Suppl):94.

158. Sultan S, Heurtier-Hartemann A. Coping and distress as predictors of glycemic control in diabetes. J Health Psychol 2001;6(6):731-9.

159. Sultan S, Luminet O, Hartemann A. Cognitive and anxiety symptoms in screening for clinical depression in diabetes A systematic examination of diagnostic performances of the HADS and BDI-SF. J Affective Disord 2010 Jun;123(1-3):332-6.

160. Suzuki A, Fujiya A, Kiyota A, Yamauchi M, et al. Approach and long-term process of a clinical network for diabetes involving a hospital which plays the central role in an area: The ogaki diabetic clinical network study. J Jpn Diabetes Soc 2007;50(5):303-11.

161. Tabaei BP, Shillnovak J, Brandle M, Burke R, et al. Glycemia and the quality of well-being in patients with diabetes. Qual Life Res 2004;13(6):1153-61.

162. Takahashi Y, Hirata Y. A follow-up study of painful diabetic neuropathy: physical and psychological aspects. Tohoku J Exp Med 1983 Dec;141(4):463-71.

163. Tapp RJ, Dunstan DW, Phillips P, Tonkin A, et al. Association between impaired glucose metabolism and quality of life: results from the Australian diabetes obesity and lifestyle study. Diabetes Res Clin Pract 2006 Nov;74(2):154-61.

164. Tsuruoka M, Yamamoto S, Tsukahara I, Akabane N, et al. A review of the low-vision clinic at Toho University Sakura Hospital. Folia Ophthalmol Jpn 2000;51(12):1131-3.

165. Upton LR. Coping with stress: Adjustment to visual loss in diabetes mellitus 1990.

166. Van Schaik HJ, itez del Castillo JM, Caubergh MJ, Gobert A, et al. Evaluation of diabetic retinopathy by fluorophotometry. European concerted action on ocular fluorometry. Int Ophthalmol 1998;22(2):97-104.

167. Varma R, Paz SH, Azen SP, Klein R, et al. The Los Angeles Latino Eye Study: design, methods, and baseline data. Ophthalmology 2004 Jun;111(6):1121-31.

168. Veglio M, Borra M, Stevens LK, Fuller JH, et al. The relation between QTc interval prolongation and diabetic complications. The EURODIAB IDDM Complication Study Group. Diabetologia 1999 Jan;42(1):68-75.

169. Vestgaard M, Ringholm L, Laugesen CS, Rasmussen KL, et al. Pregnancy-induced sight-threatening diabetic retinopathy in women with Type 1 diabetes. Diabet Med 2010 Apr;27(4):431-5.

170. Vileikyte L, Peyrot M, Gonzalez JS, Rubin RR, et al. Predictors of depressive symptoms in persons with diabetic peripheral neuropathy: A longitudinal study. Diabetologia 2009;52(7):1265-73.

171. Waldhausl W. Stimulation of immunoreactive insulin and human growth hormone release by administration of arginine in patients with diabetic retinopathy. Acta Endocrinol (Copenh) 1972;70(4):719-30.

172. Wandell PE, Tovi J. The quality of life of elderly diabetic patients. J Diabetes Complications 2000 Jan;14(1):25-30.

173. Wang C, Chan CLW, Ng S, Ho AHY. The impact of spirituality on health-related quality of life among Chinese older adults with vision impairment. Aging Ment Health 2008 Mar;12(2):267-75.

174. Warrian KJ, Lorenzana LL, Lankaranian D, Dugar J, et al. The assessment of disability related to vision performance-based measure in diabetic retinopathy. Am J Ophthalmol 2010 May;149(5):852-60.

175. Wasserman LI, Trifonova EA. Quality of Life and the Structure of Neurosis-like Symptomatology in Persons with Insulin-Dependent Diabetes Mellitus. Int J Ment Health 2004;33(3):47-57.

176. West SD, Groves DC, Lipinski HJ, Nicoll DJ, et al. The prevalence of retinopathy in men with Type 2 diabetes and obstructive sleep apnoea. Diabet Med 2010 Apr;27(4):423-30.

177. Winocour PH, Main CJ, Medlicott G, Anderson DC. A psychometric evaluation of adult patients with type 1 (insulin-dependent) diabetes mellitus: prevalence of psychological dysfunction and relationship to demographic variables, metabolic control and complications. Diabetes Res 1990 Aug;14(4):171-6.

178. Wolffsohn JS, Cochrane AL, Watt NA. Implementation methods for vision related quality of life questionnaires. Br J Ophthalmol 2000;84(9):1035-40.

179. Woodcock A, Bradley C, Plowright R, ffytche T, et al. The influence of diabetic retinopathy on quality of life: interviews to guide the design of a condition-specific, individualised questionnaire: the RetDQoL. Patient Educ Couns 2004 Jun;53(3):365-83.

180. Wulsin LR, Jacobson AM, Rand LI. Psychosocial correlates of mild visual loss. Psychosom Med 1991 Jan;53(1):109-17.

181. Wulsin LR, Jacobson AM, Rand LI. Psychosocial adjustment to advanced proliferative diabetic retinopathy. Diabetes Care 1993 Aug;16(8):1061-6.

182. Yoshida S, Hirai M, Suzuki S, Awata S, et al. Neuropathy is associated with depression independently of health-related quality of life in Japanese patients with diabetes. Psychiatry Clin Neurosci 2009 Feb;63(1):65-72.

183. Zhang CX, Tse LA, Ye XQ, Lin FY, et al. Moderating effects of coping styles on anxiety and depressive symptoms caused by psychological stress in Chinese patients with Type 2 diabetes. Diabet Med 2009;26(12):1282-8.

184. Zhao L. Intervention effects of music relaxation therapy on the quality of life in patients with diabetic retinopathy. Zhongguo Linchuang Kangfu 2005;(28):50-3.

185. Zhao W, Chen Y, Lin M, Sigal RJ. Association between diabetes and depression: Sex and age differences. Public Health 2006;120(8):696-704.

Appendix D. Characteristics of the health-related quality of life assessment tools used in studies of the treatment of diabetic retinopathy

Instrument	Administration	Domains Measured	Items/ Response Options	Scoring
Generic HRQL assessment tools				
Short Form-36 (SF–36)[56] Primary author: Ware, JE Date of 1st publication: 1992 Alternate versions: SF–36v2 (2000) Related instruments: SF–12; SF–18; SF–20;	**Target population:** general pt population, aged >14 yr **Mode of administration:** self-complete questionnaire (paper or electronic), interview, etc. **Time needed to complete:** 5–10 minutes	Physical functioning (10 items); Role limitations because of physical health problems (4 items); Bodily pain (2 items); Social functioning (2 items); General mental health (5 items); Role limitations because of emotional problems (3 items); Vitality (4 items); General health perceptions (5 items); Health transition (1 item)	**Items:** 8 items (excluding health transition); 8 scales that include 2–10 questions each; 2 summary measures, the Physical Composite Score, and the Mental Composite Score, aggregate the scales **Response options:** Items 1–3, 6–11: answered on rating scales; Item 1/2: excellent/much better to poor/much worse (5 options); Item 3: limited a lot, to not limited at all (3 options); Items 4/5: answered with a yes/no Item 6/8: not at all to extremely (5 options); Item 7: none to very severe (6 options); Item 9: all of the time to none of the time (6 options); Item 10: all of the time to none of the time (5 options); Item 11: definitely true to definitely false (5 options)	**Scoring:** each item is assigned a score on the rating scale by the pt **Final score algorithm:** items and scales were constructed for scoring using the Likert method of summated ratings **Possible range:** all scales are linearly transformed to a score between 0 (least favorable) to 100 (most favorable)

DM = diabetes mellitus; DR = diabetic retinopathy; d/t = due to; max = maximum; pt = patient; QoL: Quality of Life; r/t = related to; tx = treatment; yr = year

Appendix D. Characteristics of the health-related quality of life assessment tools used in studies of the treatment of diabetic retinopathy (continued)

Instrument	Administration	Domains Measured	Items/ Response Options	Scoring
Low vision-related HRQL assessment tools				
National Eye Institute Visual Function Questionnaire-25 (VFQ–25)[63] **Primary author:** RAND Corporation **Date of 1st publication:** 2001 **Alternate versions:** NEI-VFQ-51	**Target population:** pt with low vision **Mode of administration:** pt interview; self administered **Time needed to complete:** 5 minutes	Overall health (1 item); Overall vision (1 item); Difficulty with near vision (3 items); Difficulty with distance vision (3 items); Limitations in social functioning d/t vision (2 items); Role limitations d/t vision (2 items); Dependency on others d/t vision (3 items); Mental health symptoms d/t vision (4 items); Driving difficulties (2–3 items depending on version); Pain and discomfort around the eyes (2 items); Peripheral vision (1 item); Color vision (1 item)	**Items:** 25 or 26 items (versions vary between 2 and 3 questions in the driving domain) answer questions r/t 12 areas of visual function **Response options:** *Items 1–4:* 5 or 6-point rating scale 1 (excellent) to 5/6 (severe); *Items 5–14, 16:* 6-point rating scale 1 (no difficulty) to 5 (stopped d/t eyesight) or 6 (stopped for reason other than eyesight); *Item 15:* Yes/No; *Item 15a and 15b:* multiple choice responses; *Items 17–25:* 5-point rating scale 1 (most difficulty) to 5 (no difficulty)	**Scoring:** each item assigned a score by the pt out of 4/5/6, according to the scale used on the specific item **Final score algorithm:** *Subscales Scores:* an average of the items on each subscale transformed to a score on a 0 to 100 scale; *Composite Score:* an unweighted average of the responses to all items except for the general health rating question, which is treated as a stand-alone item **Possible range:** 0 (most severe impairment) to 100 (no impairment)
Visual Function-14 (VF-14)[66] **Primary author:** Steinberg, EP **Date of 1st publication:** 1994 **Alternate versions:** None	**Target population:** pt treated with cataract surgery **Mode of administration:** NR **Time needed to complete:** NR	Vision dependent functional activities: e.g. reading; recognizing people; seeing steps, stairs or curbs; doing fine handwork; writing checks or filling out forms; playing games, taking part in sports, cooking, watching television; and driving	**Items:** 18 questions cover 14 items **Response options:** items 1–12, 2-part questions; *Items 1-12:* Yes/No/Not Applicable; If yes, 4-point rating scale: 1 (a little difficulty)—4 (unable to do activity); *Items 13/16:* Yes/No; *Items 14/15:* 4 point rating scale: 1(no difficulty)—4 (unable to do activity); *Items 17/18:* Multiple choice responses	**Scoring:** each item is assigned a score out of 4; Score of 0 assigned when pt unable to do activity d/t visual impairment; If pt did not do activity for a reason other than vision, item not included in scoring; No min number of applicable activities required **Final score algorithm:** scores from all items pt performed or did not perform d/t their vision were averaged, resulting in a score between 0 and 4; Average score multiplied by 25 **Possible range:** 0 (most severe impairment) to100 (no impairment)

Appendix D. Characteristics of the health-related quality of life assessment tools used in studies of the treatment of diabetic retinopathy (continued)

Instrument	Administration	Domains Measured	Items/ Response Options	Scoring
Diabetes-related HRQL assessment tools				
Diabetes Treatment Satisfaction Questionnaire Status Version (DTSQs)[75] **Primary author:** Lewis, K **Date of 1st publication:** 1988 **Alternate versions:** DTSQc (change version)	**Target population:** pt with DM **Mode of administration:** self-completed questionnaire **Time needed to complete:** NR	Treatment Satisfaction (items 1, 4–8); Perceived frequency of hyperglycemia (item 2); Perceived frequency of hypoglycemia (item 3)	**Items:** 8 items **Response options:** *All items:* 7 point rating scale: 0 (very dissatisfied/none of the time) to 6 (very satisfied/most of the time);	**Scoring:** each item assigned a score by the pt out of 6 **Final score algorithm:** items, 1, 4–8 are summed to produce an overall score; Items 2 and 3 are treated individually **Possible range:** *Treatment Satisfaction:* 0 (most dissatisfied) to 36 (most satisfied); *Perceived frequency of hyperglycemia/hypoglycemia:* 0 (least frequent) to 6 (most frequent)

Appendix D. Characteristics of the health-related quality of life assessment tools used in studies of the treatment of diabetic retinopathy (continued)

Instrument	Administration	Domains Measured	Items/ Response Options	Scoring
Diabetic retinopathy-related HRQL assessment tools				
Retinopathy Dependent Quality of Life (RetDQoL)[18,70] Primary author: Woodcock, A Copyright holder: Bradley, C Date of 1st publication: 2004 Alternate versions: None	**Target population:** pt with DR **Mode of administration:** paper based questionnaire, written in a large font with a layout designed to facilitate reading by those with visual impairments **Time needed to complete:** NR	Retinopathy-dependent quality of life: e.g. household tasks; personal affairs; shopping; feelings about the future/past; working life; close personal relationship; family life; social life; do things for others; get out and about; journeys; holidays; finances; peoples reaction to me; physical appearance, physical ability; leisure; hobbies/interests; self-confidence; motivation; dependence; mishaps/losses; time; care of diabetes; enjoy nature	**Items:** overview questions: 1) present QoL; and 2) overall retinopathy-dependent QoL initiates questionnaire; Remaining 24 items r/t specific activities, which may be hindered by poor vision and affect QoL; Items 1-24 contained a part b, which assesses the importance of each item to the pt **Response options:** *Overall QoL*: 7-point rating scale: -3 (extremely bad) to 3 (excellent) *Overall DR QoL*: 5-point rating scale: -3 (very much better) to 1 (worse) *Specific domain Items 1–24*: 5-point rating scale: -3 (best/easiest) to 1 (worse/more difficult) ; *Importance ratings*: very important (3), important (2), somewhat important (1), not at all important (0) *Open-ended question*: asks whether diabetic eye problems affect QoL in any way not covered by the questionnaire	**Scoring:** *Weighted Impact score*: each specific domain is assigned an impact rating by the pt of -3 to 1 and is multiplied by the importance rating of 0 to 3, for a possible range of -9 (max negative impact) to 3 (max positive impact); Non-applicable domains are not scored **Final score algorithm:** *Average Weighted Impact score*: calculated from a max of 23 specific domain items; Sum of weighted ratings of applicable domains divided by the number of applicable domains *Note:* the 'work' items has not undergone psychometric analysis and should therefore be excluded from the average weighted impact score **Possible range:** -9 (max negative impact of DR on QoL) to 3 (max positive impact of DR on QoL)

Appendix D. Characteristics of the health-related quality of life assessment tools used in studies of the treatment of diabetic retinopathy (continued)

Instrument	Administration	Domains Measured	Items/ Response Options	Scoring
Retinopathy Treatment Satisfaction Questionnaire (RetTSQ)[71,81] Primary author: Woodcock, A Copyright holder: Bradley, C Date of 1st publication: 2005 Alternate versions: None	Target population pt with DR Mode of administration: paper based questionnaire, written in a large font with a layout designed to facilitate reading by those with visual impairments Time needed to complete: NR	Satisfaction of treatment for diabetic retinopathy: e.g. tx satisfaction, perceived effectiveness of tx; tx side effects; discomfort or pain; unpleasantness of tx; difficulty of tx; feelings of apprehension r/t tx; feelings of satisfaction regarding influence over tx; safety of tx; time-consumed by tx; information about tx; recommend tx to someone else; willingness to continue/repeat tx	Items: 13 items asking pt to rate different aspects of treatment; Items 1, 2, 8, 9, 11–13 compile the positive aspects subscale; Items 3–7 & 10 compile the negative aspects subscale Response options: 7-point rating scale: 0 (very dissatisfied/bothered/ unpleasant/difficult/apprehensive/time-consuming) to 6 (very satisfied, not at all bothered/apprehensive/unpleasant/time consuming); Open-ended question: asks respondents for any further aspects of treatment which cause satisfaction or dissatisfaction	Scoring: each item is assigned a score by the pt out of 6 Final score algorithm: *Positive aspects subscale*: calculated by summing the scores from the 7 items that make up the subscale; *Negative aspects subscale*: calculated by summing the scores from 6 items that make up the subscale *Total score*: sum of all of the 13 items that make up the RetTSQ Possible range: *Positive aspects subscale*: 0 (worst) to 42 (best); *Negative aspects subscale*: 0 (worst) to 36 (best); *Total score*: 0 (worst) to 78 (best)

Appendix E. Sample HRQL assessment tools

Generic HRQL assessment tools:
SF–36

Low vision-related HRQL assessment tools:
NEI-VFQ–25
VF–14

Diabetes-related HRQL assessment tools:
DTSQ

Diabetic retinopathy-related HRQL assessment tools:
RetDQoL
RetTSQ

Your Health and Well-Being

This survey asks for your views about your health. This information will help keep track of how you feel and how well you are able to do your usual activities. Thank you for completing this survey!

For each of the following questions, please mark an ☒ in the one box that best describes your answer.

1. In general, would you say your health is:

2. <u>Compared to one year ago</u>, how would you rate your health in general now?

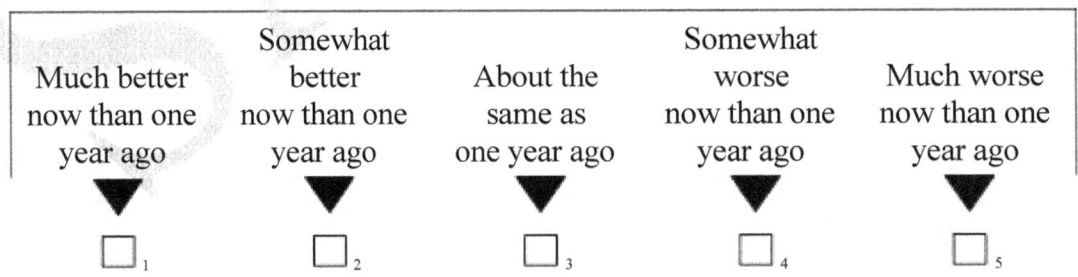

SF–36®, SF36v2®, SF–12®, and SF–12v2® are trademarks of the Medical Outcomes Trust and are used under license. The SF-25v2® Health Survey is copyrighted by QualityMetric Incorporated.

3. The following questions are about activities you might do during a typical day. Does <u>your health now limit you</u> in these activities? If so, how much?

	Yes, limited a lot ▼	Yes, limited a little ▼	No, not limited at all ▼
a <u>Vigorous activities</u>, such as running, lifting heavy objects, participating in strenuous sports	☐₁	☐₂	☐₃
b <u>Moderate activities</u>, such as moving a table, pushing a vacuum cleaner, bowling, or playing golf	☐₁	☐₂	☐₃
c Lifting or carrying groceries	☐₁	☐₂	☐₃
d Climbing <u>several</u> flights of stairs	☐₁	☐₂	☐₃
e Climbing <u>one</u> flight of stairs	☐₁	☐₂	☐₃
f Bending, kneeling, or stooping	☐₁	☐₂	☐₃
g Walking <u>more than a kilometre</u>	☐₁	☐₂	☐₃
h Walking <u>several hundred metres</u>	☐₁	☐₂	☐₃
i Walking <u>one hundred metres</u>	☐₁	☐₂	☐₃
j Bathing or dressing yourself	☐₁	☐₂	☐₃

4. During the <u>past 4 weeks</u>, how much of the time have you had any of the following problems with your work or other regular daily activities <u>as a result of your physical health</u>?

	All of the time ▼	Most of the time ▼	Some of the time ▼	A little of the time ▼	None of the time ▼
a Cut down on the <u>amount of time</u> you spent on work or other activities	☐₁	☐₂	☐₃	☐₄	☐₅
b <u>Accomplished less</u> than you would like	☐₁	☐₂	☐₃	☐₄	☐₅
c Were limited in the <u>kind</u> of work or other activities	☐₁	☐₂	☐₃	☐₄	☐₅
d Had <u>difficulty</u> performing the the work or other activities (for example, it took extra effort)	☐₁	☐₂	☐₃	☐₄	☐₅

SF–36®, SF36v2®, SF–12®, and SF–12v2® are trademarks of the Medical Outcomes Trust and are used under license. The SF-25v2® Health Survey is copyrighted by QualityMetric Incorporated.

5. During the past 4 weeks, how much of the time have you had any of the following problems with your work or other regular daily activities as a result of any emotional problems (such as feeling depressed or anxious)?

	All of the time	Most of the time	Some of the time	A little of the time	None of the time
a. Cut down on the amount of time you spent on work or other activities	☐ 1	☐ 2	☐ 3	☐ 4	☐ 5
b. Accomplished less than you would like	☐ 1	☐ 2	☐ 3	☐ 4	☐ 5
c. Did work or other activities less carefully than usual	☐ 1	☐ 2	☐ 3	☐ 4	☐ 5

6. During the past 4 weeks, to what extent has your physical health or emotional problems interfered with your normal social activities with family, friends, neighbors, or groups?

Not at all	Slightly	Moderately	Quite a bit	Extremely
☐ 1	☐ 2	☐ 3	☐ 4	☐ 5

7. How much bodily pain have you had during the past 4 weeks?

None	Very mild	Mild	Moderate	Severe	Very severe
☐ 1	☐ 2	☐ 3	☐ 4	☐ 5	☐ 6

SF–36®, SF36v2®, SF–12®, and SF–12v2® are trademarks of the Medical Outcomes Trust and are used under license. The SF-25v2® Health Survey is copyrighted by QualityMetric Incorporated.

8. During the past 4 weeks, how much did pain interfere with your normal work (including both work outside the home and housework)?

Not at all	A little bit	Moderately	Quite a bit	Extremely
▼	▼	▼	▼	▼
☐₁	☐₂	☐₃	☐₄	☐₅

9. These questions are about how you feel and how things have been with you during the past 4 weeks. For each question, please give the one answer that comes closest to the way you have been feeling. How much of the time during the past 4 weeks…

	All of the time	Most of the time	Some of the time	A little of the time	None of the time
a Did you feel full of life?	☐₁	☐₂	☐₃	☐₄	☐₅
b Have you been very nervous?	☐₁	☐₂	☐₃	☐₄	☐₅
c Have you felt so down in the dumps that nothing could cheer you up?	☐₁	☐₂	☐₃	☐₄	☐₅
d Have you felt calm and peaceful?	☐₁	☐₂	☐₃	☐₄	☐₅
e Did you have a lot of energy?	☐₁	☐₂	☐₃	☐₄	☐₅
f Have you felt downhearted and depressed?	☐₁	☐₂	☐₃	☐₄	☐₅
g Did you feel worn out?	☐₁	☐₂	☐₃	☐₄	☐₅
h Have you been happy?	☐₁	☐₂	☐₃	☐₄	☐₅
i Did you feel tired?	☐₁	☐₂	☐₃	☐₄	☐₅

SF–36®, SF36v2®, SF–12®, and SF–12v2® are trademarks of the Medical Outcomes Trust and are used under license. The SF-25v2® Health Survey is copyrighted by QualityMetric Incorporated.

10. During the past 4 weeks, how much of the time has your physical health or emotional problems interfered with your social activities (like visiting with friends, relatives, etc.)?

All of the time	Most of the time	Some of the time	A little of the time	None of the time
▼	▼	▼	▼	▼
☐₁	☐₂	☐₃	☐₄	☐₅

11. How TRUE or FALSE is each of the following statements for you?

		Definitely true ▼	Mostly true ▼	Don't know ▼	Mostly false ▼	Definitely false ▼
a	I seem to get sick a little easier than other people	☐₁	☐₂	☐₃	☐₄	☐₅
b	I am as healthy as anybody I know	☐₁	☐₂	☐₃	☐₄	☐₅
c	I expect my health to get worse	☐₁	☐₂	☐₃	☐₄	☐₅
d	My health is excellent	☐₁	☐₂	☐₃	☐₄	☐₅

Thank you for completing these questions!

SF–36®, SF36v2®, SF–12®, and SF–12v2® are trademarks of the Medical Outcomes Trust and are used under license. The SF–25v2® Health Survey is copyrighted by QualityMetric Incorporated.

PB/SA

National Eye Institute
Visual Functioning Questionnaire - 25
(VFQ-25)

version 2000

(SELF-ADMINISTERED FORMAT)

January 2000

RAND hereby grants permission to use the "National Eye Institute Visual Functioning Questionnaire 25 (VFQ-25) July 1996, in accordance with the following conditions which shall be assumed by all to have been agreed to as a consequence of accepting and using this document:

1. Changes to the NEI VFQ-25 - July 1996 may be made without the written permission of RAND. However, all such changes shall be clearly identified as having been made by the recipient.

2. The user of this NEI VFQ-25 - July 1996 accepts full responsibility, and agrees to hold RAND harmless, for the accuracy of any translations of the NEI VFQ-25 Test Version - July 1996 into another language and for any errors, omissions, misinterpretations, or consequences thereof.

3. The user of this NEI VFQ-25 - July 1996 accepts full responsibility, and agrees to hold RAND harmless, for any consequences resulting from the use of the NEI VFQ-25.

4. The user of the NEI VFQ-25 - July 1996 will provide a credit line when printing and distributing this document or in publications of results or analyses based on this instrument acknowledging that it was developed at RAND under the sponsorship of the National Eye Institute.

5. No further written permission is needed for use of this NEI VFQ-25 - July 1996.

7/29/96

© RAND 1996

version 2000

The following is a survey with statements about problems which involve your vision or feelings that you have about your vision condition. After each question please choose the response that best describes your situation.

Please answer all the questions as if you were wearing your glasses or contact lenses (if any).

Please take as much time as you need to answer each question. All your answers are confidential. In order for this survey to improve our knowledge about vision problems and how they affect your quality of life, your answers must be as accurate as possible. Remember, if you wear glasses or contact lenses, please answer all of the following questions as though you were wearing them.

INSTRUCTIONS:

1. In general we would like to have people try to complete these forms on their own. If you find that you need assistance, please feel free to ask the project staff and they will assist you.

2. Please answer every question (unless you are asked to skip questions because they don't apply to you).

3. Answer the questions by circling the appropriate number.

4. If you are unsure of how to answer a question, please give the best answer you can and make a comment in the left margin.

5. Please complete the questionnaire before leaving the center and give it to a member of the project staff. Do not take it home.

6. If you have any questions, please feel free to ask a member of the project staff, and they will be glad to help you.

STATEMENT OF CONFIDENTIALITY:

All information that would permit identification of any person who completed this questionnaire will be regarded as strictly confidential. Such information will be used only for the purposes of this study and will not be disclosed or released for any other purposes without prior consent, except as required by law.

© **RAND** 1996

version 2000

Visual Functioning Questionnaire - 25

PART 1 - GENERAL HEALTH AND VISION

1. <u>In general,</u> would you say your overall <u>health</u> is:

    (Circle One)

Excellent	1
Very Good	2
Good	3
Fair	4
Poor	5

2. At the present time, would you say your eyesight using both eyes (with glasses or contact lenses, if you wear them) is <u>excellent</u>, <u>good</u>, <u>fair</u>, <u>poor</u>, or <u>very poor</u> or are you <u>completely blind</u>?

    (Circle One)

Excellent	1
Good	2
Fair	3
Poor	4
Very Poor	5
Completely Blind	6

© **RAND** 1996

3. How much of the time do you worry about your eyesight?

	(Circle One)
None of the time	1
A little of the time	2
Some of the time	3
Most of the time	4
All of the time?	5

4. How much pain or discomfort have you had in and around your eyes (for example, burning, itching, or aching)? Would you say it is:

	(Circle One)
None	1
Mild	2
Moderate	3
Severe, or	4
Very severe?	5

PART 2 - DIFFICULTY WITH ACTIVITIES

The next questions are about how much difficulty, if any, you have doing certain activities wearing your glasses or contact lenses if you use them for that activity.

5. How much difficulty do you have reading ordinary print in newspapers? Would you say you have:

	(Circle One)
No difficulty at all	1
A little difficulty	2
Moderate difficulty	3
Extreme difficulty	4
Stopped doing this because of your eyesight	5
Stopped doing this for other reasons or not interested in doing this	6

© RAND 1996

6. How much difficulty do you have doing work or hobbies that require you to <u>see well up close</u>, such as cooking, sewing, fixing things around the house, or using hand tools? Would you say:

                                                                                            (Circle One)

    No difficulty at all 1
    A little difficulty 2
    Moderate difficulty 3
    Extreme difficulty 4
    Stopped doing this because of your eyesight 5
    Stopped doing this for other reasons or not
        interested in doing this 6

7. Because of your eyesight, how much difficulty do you have <u>finding something on a crowded shelf</u>?

                                                                                            (Circle One)

    No difficulty at all 1
    A little difficulty 2
    Moderate difficulty 3
    Extreme difficulty 4
    Stopped doing this because of your eyesight 5
    Stopped doing this for other reasons or not
        interested in doing this 6

8. How much difficulty do you have <u>reading street signs or the names of stores</u>?

                                                                                            (Circle One)

    No difficulty at all 1
    A little difficulty 2
    Moderate difficulty 3
    Extreme difficulty 4
    Stopped doing this because of your eyesight 5
    Stopped doing this for other reasons or not
        interested in doing this 6

9. Because of your eyesight, how much difficulty do you have <u>going down steps, stairs, or curbs in dim light or at night</u>?

	(Circle One)
No difficulty at all	1
A little difficulty	2
Moderate difficulty	3
Extreme difficulty	4
Stopped doing this because of your eyesight	5
Stopped doing this for other reasons or not interested in doing this	6

10. Because of your eyesight, how much difficulty do you have <u>noticing objects off to the side while you are walking along</u>?

	(Circle One)
No difficulty at all	1
A little difficulty	2
Moderate difficulty	3
Extreme difficulty	4
Stopped doing this because of your eyesight	5
Stopped doing this for other reasons or not interested in doing this	6

11. Because of your eyesight, how much difficulty do you have <u>seeing how people react to things</u> you say?

	(Circle One)
No difficulty at all	1
A little difficulty	2
Moderate difficulty	3
Extreme difficulty	4
Stopped doing this because of your eyesight	5
Stopped doing this for other reasons or not interested in doing this	6

© **RAND** 1996

12. Because of your eyesight, how much difficulty do you have <u>picking out and matching your own clothes</u>?

                                                                                       (Circle One)

- No difficulty at all 1
- A little difficulty 2
- Moderate difficulty 3
- Extreme difficulty 4
- Stopped doing this because of your eyesight 5
- Stopped doing this for other reasons or not interested in doing this 6

13. Because of your eyesight, how much difficulty do you have <u>visiting with people in their homes, at parties, or in restaurants</u>?

                                                                                       (Circle One)

- No difficulty at all 1
- A little difficulty 2
- Moderate difficulty 3
- Extreme difficulty 4
- Stopped doing this because of your eyesight 5
- Stopped doing this for other reasons or not interested in doing this 6

14. Because of your eyesight, how much difficulty do you have <u>going out to see movies, plays, or sports events</u>?

                                                                                       (Circle One)

- No difficulty at all 1
- A little difficulty 2
- Moderate difficulty 3
- Extreme difficulty 4
- Stopped doing this because of your eyesight 5
- Stopped doing this for other reasons or not interested in doing this 6

15. Are you <u>currently driving</u>, at least once in a while?

© **RAND** 1996

(Circle One)

Yes .... 1 Skip To Q 15c

No 2

15a. IF NO: Have you <u>never driven a car or have you given up driving</u>?

(Circle One)

Never drove ...... 1 Skip To Part 3, Q 17

Gave up 2

15b. IF YOU GAVE UP DRIVING: Was that <u>mainly because of your eyesight</u>, <u>mainly for some other reason</u>, or <u>because of both your eyesight and other reasons</u>?

(Circle One)

Mainly eyesight .... 1 Skip To Part 3, Q 17

Mainly other reasons .... 2 Skip To Part 3, Q 17

Both eyesight and other reasons .... 3 Skip To Part 3, Q 17

15c. IF CURRENTLY DRIVING: How much difficulty do you have <u>driving during the daytime in familiar places</u>? Would you say you have:

(Circle One)

No difficulty at all.............................. 1
A little difficulty................................ 2
Moderate difficulty............................ 3
Extreme difficulty 4

© RAND 1996

16. How much difficulty do you have <u>driving at night</u>? Would you say you have:

	(Circle One)
No difficulty at all	1
A little difficulty	2
Moderate difficulty	3
Extreme difficulty	4
Have you stopped doing this because of your eyesight	5
Have you stopped doing this for other reasons or are you not interested in doing this	6

16A. How much difficulty do you have <u>driving in difficult conditions, such as in bad weather, during rush hour, on the freeway, or in city traffic</u>? Would you say you have:

	(Circle One)
No difficulty at all	1
A little difficulty	2
Moderate difficulty	3
Extreme difficulty	4
Have you stopped doing this because of your eyesight	5
Have you stopped doing this for other reasons or are you not interested in doing this	6

© RAND 1996

PART 3: RESPONSES TO VISION PROBLEMS

The next questions are about how things you do may be affected by your vision. For each one, please circle the number to indicate whether for you the statement is true for you <u>all</u>, <u>most</u>, <u>some</u>, <u>a little</u>, or <u>none</u> of the time.

(Circle One On Each Line)

READ CATEGORIES:	All of the time	Most of the time	Some of the time	A little of the time	None of the time
17. <u>Do you accomplish less</u> than you would like because of your vision?	1	2	3	4	5
18. <u>Are you limited</u> in how long you can work or do other activities because of your vision?	1	2	3	4	5
19. How much does pain or discomfort <u>in or around your eyes</u>, for example, burning, itching, or aching, keep you from doing what you'd like to be doing? Would you say:	1	2	3	4	5

© **RAND** 1996

For each of the following statements, please circle the number to indicate whether for you the statement is <u>definitely true</u>, <u>mostly true</u>, <u>mostly false</u>, or <u>definitely false</u> for you or you are <u>not sure</u>.

(Circle One On Each Line)

	Definitely True	Mostly True	Not Sure	Mostly False	Definitely False
20. I <u>stay home most of the time</u> because of my eyesight	1	2	3	4	5
21. I feel <u>frustrated</u> a lot of the time because of my eyesight	1	2	3	4	5
22. I have <u>much less control</u> over what I do, because of my eyesight	1	2	3	4	5
23. Because of my eyesight, I have to <u>rely too much on what other people tell me</u>	1	2	3	4	5
24. I <u>need a lot of help</u> from others because of my eyesight	1	2	3	4	5
25. I worry about <u>doing things that will embarrass myself or others</u>, because of my eyesight	1	2	3	4	5

© **RAND** 1996

version 2000

Appendix of Optional Additional Questions

SUBSCALE: GENERAL HEALTH

A1. How would you rate your <u>overall health, on a scale where zero is as bad as death</u> and 10 is <u>best</u> possible health?

(Circle One)

0   1   2   3   4   5   6   7   8   9   10
Worst   Best

SUBSCALE: GENERAL VISION

A2. How would you rate your eyesight now (with glasses or contact lens on, if you wear them), on a scale of from 0 to 10, where zero means the worst possible eyesight, as bad or worse than being blind, and 10 means the best possible eyesight?

(Circle One)

0   1   2   3   4   5   6   7   8   9   10
Worst   Best

SUBSCALE: NEAR VISION

A3. Wearing glasses, how much difficulty do you have <u>reading the small print in a telephone book, on a medicine bottle, or on legal forms</u>? Would you say:

(Circle One)

No difficulty at all	1
A little difficulty	2
Moderate difficulty	3
Extreme difficulty	4
Stopped doing this because of your eyesight	5
Stopped doing this for other reasons or not interested in doing this	6

© **RAND** 1996

A4. Because of your eyesight, how much difficulty do you have <u>figuring out whether bills you receive are accurate</u>?

	(Circle One)
No difficulty at all	1
A little difficulty	2
Moderate difficulty	3
Extreme difficulty	4
Stopped doing this because of your eyesight	5
Stopped doing this for other reasons or not interested in doing this	6

A5. Because of your eyesight, how much difficulty do you have doing things like <u>shaving, styling your hair, or putting on makeup</u>?

	(Circle One)
No difficulty at all	1
A little difficulty	2
Moderate difficulty	3
Extreme difficulty	4
Stopped doing this because of your eyesight	5
Stopped doing this for other reasons or not interested in doing this	6

SUBSCALE: DISTANCE VISION

A6. Because of your eyesight, how much difficulty do you have <u>recognizing people you know from across a room</u>?

	(Circle One)
No difficulty at all	1
A little difficulty	2
Moderate difficulty	3
Extreme difficulty	4
Stopped doing this because of your eyesight	5
Stopped doing this for other reasons or not interested in doing this	6

© **RAND** 1996

A7. Because of your eyesight, how much difficulty do you have <u>taking part in active sports or other outdoor activities that you enjoy</u> (like golf, bowling, jogging, or walking)?

	(Circle One)
No difficulty at all	1
A little difficulty	2
Moderate difficulty	3
Extreme difficulty	4
Stopped doing this because of your eyesight	5
Stopped doing this for other reasons or not interested in doing this	6

A8. Because of your eyesight, how much difficulty do you have <u>seeing and enjoying programs on TV</u>?

	(Circle One)
No difficulty at all	1
A little difficulty	2
Moderate difficulty	3
Extreme difficulty	4
Stopped doing this because of your eyesight	5
Stopped doing this for other reasons or not interested in doing this	6

SUBSCALE: SOCIAL FUNCTION

A9. Because of your eyesight, how much difficulty do you have <u>entertaining friends and family in your home</u>?

	(Circle One)
No difficulty at all	1
A little difficulty	2
Moderate difficulty	3
Extreme difficulty	4
Stopped doing this because of your eyesight	5
Stopped doing this for other reasons or not interested in doing this	6

© RAND 1996

SUBSCALE: DRIVING

A10. [This item, "driving in difficult conditions", has been included as part of the base set of 25 items as item 16a.]

SUBSCALE: ROLE LIMITATIONS

A11. The next questions are about things you may do because of your vision. For each item, please circle the number to indicate whether for you this is true for you <u>all</u>, <u>most</u>, <u>some</u>, <u>a little</u>, or <u>none</u> of the time.

(Circle One On Each Line)

	All of the time	Most of the time	Some of the time	A little of the time	None of the time
a. <u>Do you have more help</u> from others because of your vision?	1	2	3	4	5
b. <u>Are you limited</u> in the kinds of things you can do because of your vision?	1	2	3	4	5

© **RAND** 1996

SUBSCALES: WELL-BEING/DISTRESS (#A12) and DEPENDENCY (#A13)

The next questions are about how you deal with your vision. For each statement, please circle the number to indicate whether for you it is definitely true, mostly true, mostly false, or definitely false for you or you don't know.

(Circle One On Each Line)

	Definitely True	Mostly True	Not Sure	Mostly False	Definitely False
A12. I am often irritable because of my eyesight	1	2	3	4	5
A13. I don't go out of my home alone, because of my eyesight	1	2	3	4	5

© **RAND** 1996

Visual Function—14 Questionnaire

1. Do you have any difficulty, even with glasses, reading small print, such as labels on medicine bottles, a telephone book, food labels?
__ Yes __ No __ Not applicable
If yes, how much difficulty do you currently have?
1. A little
2. A moderate amount
3. A great deal
4. Are you unable to do the activity?

2. Do you have any difficulty, even with glasses, reading a newspaper or a book?
__ Yes __ No __ Not applicable
If yes, how much difficulty do you currently have?
1. A little
2. A moderate amount
3. A great deal
4. Are you unable to do the activity?

3. Do you have any difficulty, even with glasses, reading a large-print book or large-print newspaper or numbers on a telephone?
__ Yes __ No __ Not applicable
If yes, how much difficulty do you currently have?
1. A little
2. A moderate amount
3. A great deal
4. Are you unable to do the activity?

4. Do you have difficulty, even with glasses, recognizing people when they are close to you?
__ Yes __ No __ Not applicable
If yes, how much difficulty do you currently have?
1. A little
2. A moderate amount
3. A great deal
4. Are you unable to do the activity?

5. Do you have difficulty, even with glasses, seeing steps, stairs or curbs?
__ Yes __ No __ Not applicable
If yes, how much difficulty do you currently have?
1. A little
2. A moderate amount
3. A great deal
4. Are you unable to do the activity?

6. Do you have any difficulty, even with glasses, reading traffic signs, street signs, or store signs?
__ Yes __ No __ Not applicable
If yes, how much difficulty do you currently have?
1. A little
2. A moderate amount
3. A great deal
4. Are you unable to do the activity?

7. Do you have any difficulty, even with glasses, doing fine handwork like sewing, knitting, crocheting, carpentry?
__ Yes __ No __ Not applicable
If yes, how much difficulty do you currently have?
1. A little
2. A moderate amount
3. A great deal
4. Are you unable to do the activity?

8. Do you have any difficulty, even with glasses, writing checks or filling out forms?
__ Yes __ No __ Not applicable
If yes, how much difficulty do you currently have?
1. A little
2. A moderate amount
3. A great deal
4. Are you unable to do the activity?

9. Do you have any difficulty, even with glasses, playing games such as bingo, dominos, card games, mahjong?
__ Yes __ No __ Not applicable
If yes, how much difficulty do you currently have?
1. A little
2. A moderate amount
3. A great deal
4. Are you unable to do the activity?

10. Do you have any difficulty, even with glasses, taking part in sports like bowling, handball, tennis, golf?
__ Yes __ No __ Not applicable
If yes, how much difficulty do you currently have?
1. A little
2. A moderate amount
3. A great deal
4. Are you unable to do the activity?

11. Do you have any difficulty, even with glasses, cooking?
__ Yes __ No __ Not applicable
If yes, how much difficulty do you currently have?
1. A little
2. A moderate amount
3. A great deal
4. Are you unable to do the activity?

12. Do you have any difficulty, even with glasses, watching television?
__ Yes __ No __ Not applicable
If yes, how much difficulty do you currently have?
1. A little
2. A moderate amount
3. A great deal
4. Are you unable to do the activity?

13. Do you currently drive a car?
__ Yes (go to 14) __ No (go to 16)

14. How much difficulty do you have driving during the day because of your vision? Do you have:
1. No difficulty
2. A little difficulty
3. A moderate amount of difficulty
4. A great deal of difficulty?

15. How much difficulty do you have driving at night because of your vision? Do you have:
1. No difficulty
2. A little difficulty
3. A moderate amount of difficulty
4. A great deal of difficulty?

16. Have you ever driven a car?
__ Yes (go to 17) __ No (stop)

17. When did you stop driving?
__ Less than 6 months ago
__ 6–12 months ago
__ More than 12 months ago

18. Why did you stop driving?
__ Vision
__ Other illness
__ Other reason

Reprinted with permission: Steinberg EP, Tielsch JM, Schein OD, et al. The VF–14. An index of functional impairment in patients with cataract. Arch Ophthalmol 1994;112:630–638.

Items included in the Diabetes Treatment Satisfaction Questionnaire (DTSQ)

The following questions are concerned with the treatment of your diabetes (including insulin, tablets and/or diet) and your experience over the past few weeks.

#	Question	Scale
1	How satisfied are you with your current treatment?	very satisfied — very dissatisfied
2	How often have you felt that your blood sugars have been unacceptably high recently?	most of the time — none of the time
3	How often have you felt that your blood sugars have been unacceptably low recently?	most of the time — none of the time
4	How convenient have you been finding your treatment to be recently?	very convenient — very inconvenient
5	How flexible have you been finding your treatment to be recently?	very flexible — very inflexible
6	How satisfied are you with your understanding of your diabetes?	very satisfied — very dissatisfied
7	Would you recommend this form of treatment to someone else with your kind of diabetes?	yes, I would definitely recommend the treatment — no, I would definitely not recommend the treatment
8	How satisfied would you be to continue with your present form of treatment?	very satisfied — very dissatisfied

Reprinted with permission: Prof. Clare Bradley, Health Psychology Research, University of London, Egham, Surrey, TW20 OEX, UK

Items included in the Retinopathy Dependent Quality of Life (RetDQoL) Questionnaire

	This questionnaire asks about your quality of life—in other words, how good or bad you feel your life is.	
I	In general, my present quality of life is:	excellent — extremely bad
II	If I did not have diabetic eye problems, my quality of life would be:	very much better — worse
	NOTE: All items 1–24 begin with the phrase: If I did not have diabetic eye problems:	
1	I could handle my household tasks:	very much better — worse
2	I could handle my personal affairs (letters, bills, etc):	very much better — worse
3	My experience of shopping would be:	very much better — worse
4	My feelings about the future (e.g. worries, hopes) would be:	very much better — worse
5	My feelings about past medical care and/or self-care (e.g. anger or regret) would be:	very much better — worse
6	*My work life would be:	very much better — worse
7	*My closest personal relationship would be:	very much better — worse
8	*If I did not have diabetic eye problems, my family life would be:	very much better — worse
9	My friendships and social life would be:	very much better — worse
10	I could do things for others as I wish:	very much better — worse
11	I could get out and about (e.g. on foot, or by car, bus or train):	very much better — worse
12	*My vacations would be:	very much better — worse
13	My financial situation would be:	very much better — worse
14	The way people in general react to me would be:	very much better — worse
15	My physical appearance (including clothes and grooming) would be:	very much better — worse
16	Physically I could do:	very much more — less
17	I could enjoy my leisure activities and interests (e.g. reading, TV, radio, hobbies):	very much more — less
18	My self-confidence would be:	very much better — worse
19	My motivation would be:	very much better — worse
20	*I could do things independently:	very much better — worse
21	I would have mishaps or would lose things:	very much less — more
22	The time it takes me to do things would be:	very much less — more
23	I would find taking care of my diabetes (e.g. self-testing, medication, food, exercise):	very much easier — more difficult
24	I could enjoy nature:	very much more — less
25	Do your diabetic eye problems affect your quality of life in any ways that have not been covered by the questionnaire?	If 'yes', please describe.

*Denotes a 'not applicable' option

Reprinted with permission: Prof. Clare Bradley, Health Psychology Research, University of London, Egham, Surrey, TW20 OEX, UK

Content of the 2 overview items (showing the scores assigned)

I) In general, my present quality of life is:	
Excellent	3
Very good	2
Good	1
Neither good nor bad	0
Bad	-1
Very bad	-2
Extremely bad	-3

II) If I did not have diabetic eye problems, my quality of life would be:	
Very much better	-3
Much better	-2
A little better	-1
The same	0
Worse	1

Content of a condition-specific domain (showing the scores assigned)

9a) If I did not have diabetic eye problems, my friendships and social life would be:	
Very much better	-3
Much better	-2
A little better	-1
The same	0
Worse	1

9b) My friendships and social life are:	
Very important	3
Important	2
Somewhat important	1
Not at all important	0

Items included in the Retinopathy Treatment Satisfaction Questionnaire (RetTSQ)

The following questions are about your experience of treatment for your diabetic eye problems—the eye problems often caused by diabetes

1	How satisfied are you with the treatment for your diabetic eye problems?	very satisfied — very dissatisfied
2	How well do you feel the treatment for your diabetic eye problems is working?	very well — very badly
3	How bothered are you by any side effects both during and after treatment for your diabetic eye problems?	not at all bothered — very bothered
4	How bothered are you by any discomfort or pain from the treatment for your diabetic eye problems?	not at all bothered — very bothered
5	How unpleasant do you find the treatment for your diabetic eye problems?	not at all unpleasant — very unpleasant
6	How difficult for you is the treatment for your diabetic eye problems?	very easy — very difficult
7	How apprehensive do you feel about the treatment for your diabetic eye problems?	not at all apprehensive — very apprehensive
8	How satisfied are you with the influence you have over the treatment for your diabetic eye problems?	very satisfied — very dissatisfied
9	How satisfied are you with the safety of the treatment for your diabetic eye problems?	very satisfied — very dissatisfied
10	How satisfied are you with the time taken by the treatment for your diabetic eye problems?	very satisfied — very dissatisfied
11	How satisfied are you with the information provided about the treatment for your diabetic eye problems?	very satisfied — very dissatisfied
12	Would you encourage someone else with diabetic eye problems like yours to have a treatment similar to yours?	yes, I would definitely encourage them — no, I would definitely not encourage them
13	How satisfied would you be to continue or repeat the treatment for your diabetic eye problems?	very satisfied — very dissatisfied
14	Are there any other features of the treatment for your diabetic eye problems, causing you either satisfaction or dissatisfaction, that have not been covered by the questionnaire?	If 'yes', please describe.

Reprinted with permission: Prof. Clare Bradley, Health Psychology Research, University of London, Egham, Surrey, TW20 OEX, UK

Appendix F. Extended study characteristics and outcomes for studies reporting the impact of interventions for diabetic retinopathy on HRQL

Study	Study Characteristics	Study Population	HRQL Instrument(s)	Results
Laser photocoagulation				
Tranos, 2004[44] **Country:** UK **Date of study:** February 2001 to August 2002 **Study setting:** outpatient clinic	**Study design:** prospective cohort **Inclusion criteria:** 1) age ≥17 yr; 2) English speaking; 3) evidence of DME by slit lamp biomicroscopy; 4) pass on an abbreviated version of the Folstein Mini-Mental State examination **Exclusion criteria:** 1) previous laser photocoagulation for PDR or DME 2) vitreous hemorrhage present at recruitment or after enrollment; 3) clinically significant coexisting ocular pathology such as glaucoma and ARMD **Intervention (n):** G1 (all pt)—laser tx; focal laser tx (38), grid laser tx (17)	**Total population (n):** 64 **Total eyes in study (n):** NR **Withdrew (n):** developed vitreous hemorrhage (2), proliferative diabetic changes requiring panretinal photocoagulation (4), moved and had ongoing follow-up by a non study ophthalmologist (3) **Analyzed n (%):** 55 (85.9) **Age, mean±SD(range):** 65.1±9.7 (NR) **Males n (%):** 17 (30.9) **Type of DM n (%):** NR **Visual acuity:** NR **DR n (%):** 55 (100) **DME n (%):** 55 (100) **Type of DR n (%):** mild NPDR—13 (23.6); moderate NPDR—32 (58.2); severe NPDR—10 (18.2)	**Instrument/technique:** NEI-VFQ-51 **Method of administration:** pt self-completed with verbal instructions and assistance from research staff **Respondent:** Pt **Time points of administration:** before and 3–4 mo after tx **Baseline score mean±SD(range):** NEI-VFQ-51 G1—77.9 (17.6)	*VFQ-51 composite score*—82.8 ±15.1 improvement: 4.9±8.9 (p < 0.001) *Subscales*—statistically significant improvement on 8 of 11 vision-related domains *Distance vision*—baseline: 42.7±8.4 letters; improvement: 2.2±6.2 *Near vision*—baseline: 56.4±9.1 letters; improvement: 2.1±5.0

ARMD = age-related macular degeneration; BCVA = best corrected visual acuity; BRVO = branch retinal vein occlusion; CRVO = central retinal vein occlusion; CS = contrast sensitivity; DM = diabetes mellitus; DME = diabetic macular edema; DR = diabetic retinopathy; Diabetes Treatment Satisfaction Questionnaire = DTSQ; ERM = epiretinal membrane; ETDRS = Early Treatment Diabetic Retinopathy Research Group; hx = history; LTF = lost to followup; MH = macular hole; mo = month; NPDR = non proliferative diabetic retinopathy; NR = not reported; OCT = optical coherence tomography; PDR = proliferative diabetic retinopathy; pt = patient; QOL = quality of life; RD = rhegmatogenous retinal detachment; RBX = Ruboxistaurin; T1D = type 1 diabetes mellitus; T2D = type 2 diabetes mellitus; tx = treatment; VA = visual acuity; VF = visual function; VFQ-25 = National Eye Institute Visual Function Questionnaire-25; yr = year(s)

Appendix F. Extended study characteristics and outcomes for studies reporting the impact of interventions for diabetic retinopathy on HRQL (continued)

Study	Study Characteristics	Study Population	HRQL Instrument(s)	Results
Mozaffarieh, 2005b[50] **Country:** Austria **Date of study:** June 2002 to March 2004 **Study setting:** outpatient clinic	**Study design:** prospective cohort **Inclusion criteria:** 1) undergoing 1st laser tx for DME or PDR **Exclusion criteria:** NR **Intervention (n):** G1—pt with PDR: panretinal photocoagulation tx for neovascularization on the disk, or elsewhere in accordance to ETDRS guidelines (56); G2—pt with DME: macular laser tx, as defined by ETDRS guidelines for retinal edema threatening the fovea (49)	**Total population (n):** 123 **Total eyes in study (n):** **Withdrew (n):** died (2), LTF (3), did not complete/return questionnaire (13) **Analyzed n (%):** 105 (85.4) **Age, mean±SD(range):** NR **Males n (%):** NR **Type of DM n (%):** NR **Visual acuity:** NR **DR n (%):** 56 (53.3) **Type of DR n (%):** PDR—56 (53.3) **DME n (%):** 49 (46.7)	**Instrument/technique:** DTSQ; Degree of satisfaction (questionnaire developed for study) **Respondent:** Pt **Time points of administration:** *DTSQ*—after initial tx (baseline) and final (9 mo.) tx; *Degree of satisfaction*—after final (9 mo.) tx **Baseline score mean±SD(range):** *DTSQ*—29.6±5.6; 45.7% of all pt scored ≥31 (max 36); for 5 of 6 subscales, 59.1% of pt scores ≥25	*DTSQ (mean±SD)*—27.9±5.2 *Degree of satisfaction*—69.5% of pt completely satisfied, 20.9% partially satisfied, 9.6% dissatisfied *Patient reported VA*—24.7% of all pt reported improvement in VA; 71.4% of pt reported no change in VA; 3.8% of pt reported deterioration in VA

ARMD = age-related macular degeneration; BCVA = best corrected visual acuity; BRVO = branch retinal vein occlusion; CRVO = central retinal vein occlusion; CS = contrast sensitivity; DM = diabetes mellitus; DME = diabetic macular edema; DR = diabetic retinopathy; Diabetes Treatment Satisfaction Questionnaire = DTSQ; ERM = epiretinal membrane; ETDRS = Early Treatment Diabetic Retinopathy Research Group; hx = history; LTF = lost to followup; MH = macular hole; mo = month; NPDR = non proliferative diabetic retinopathy; NR = not reported; OCT = optical coherence tomography; PDR = proliferative diabetic retinopathy; pt = patient; QOL = quality of life; RD = rhegmatogenous retinal detachment; RBX = Ruboxistaurin; T1D = type 1 diabetes mellitus; T2D = type 2 diabetes mellitus; tx = treatment; VA = visual acuity; VF = visual function; VFQ-25 = National Eye Institute Visual Function Questionnaire-25; yr = year(s)

Appendix F. Extended study characteristics and outcomes for studies reporting the impact of interventions for diabetic retinopathy on HRQL (continued)

Study	Study Characteristics	Study Population	HRQL Instrument(s)	Results
Vitrectomy				
Emi, 2008[72]	Study design: cohort	Total population (n): 87	Instrument/technique: VFQ–25	VFQ–25 6 mo scores per item (mean):
	Inclusion criteria: 1) Pt dx with DR; 2) Pt who underwent vitrectomy	Total eyes in study (n): 87	Respondent: Pt	G1—Item 1: 39; Item 2: 68; Item 3: 91; Item 4: 70; Item 5: 77; Item 6: 87; Item 7: 74; Item 8: 78; Item 9: 79; Item 10: 68; Item 11: 95; Item 12: 80
Country: Japan		Withdrew (n): 0 (0)		
Date of study: NR		Analyzed n (%): 87 (100%)	Time points of administration: VFQ–25 baseline; 6 mo after tx	
Study setting: NR	Exclusion criteria: NR	Age, mean±SD(range):		G2—Item 1: 42; Item 2: 53; Item 3: 94; Item 4: 58; Item 5: 72; Item 6: 79; Item 7: 65; Item 8: 73; Item 9: 80; Item 10: 58; Item 11: 91; Item 12: 79
	Intervention (n):	G1—60.4 (7.1)	Baseline score mean±SD(range):	
	All groups—pars plana vitrectomy (87)	G2—63.6 (5.0)	VFQ–25, scores per item:	
		G3—55.3 (9.0)		G3—Item 1: 45; Item 2: 63; Item 3: 80; Item 4: 66; Item 5: 75; Item 6: 87; Item 7: 66; Item 8: 72; Item 9: 75; Item 10: 52; Item 11: 95; Item 12: 80
		Males n (%):	G1—Item 1: 37; Item 2: 42; Item 3: 94; Item 4: 47; Item 5: 58; Item 6: 75; Item 7: 54; Item 8: 62; Item 9: 69; Item 10: 35; Item 11: 89; Item 12: 65;	
	Patient groups n (%)	G1—23 (56.1)		
	G1—vitreous hemorrhage: 41 (47.1);	G2—18 (64.3)		
	G2—DME: 28 (32.2);	G3—9 (50)		
	G3—fibrovascular membrane: 18 (20.7)	Type of DM n (%): NR	G2—Item 1: 42; Item 2: 45; Item 3: 93; Item 4: 57; Item 5: 71; Item 6: 86; Item 7: 64; Item 8: 78; Item 9: 81; Item 10: 54; Item 11: 96; Item 12: 77;	
		Visual acuity: NR		
		DR n (%): 87 (100%)	G3—Item 1: 45; Item 2: 47; Item 3: 93; Item 4: 74; Item 5: 83; Item 6: 93; Item 7: 72; Item 8: 79; Item 9: 89; Item 10: 51; Item 11: 87; Item 12: 85	
		Type of DR n (%): NR		

ARMD = age-related macular degeneration; BCVA = best corrected visual acuity; BRVO = branch retinal vein occlusion; CRVO = central retinal vein occlusion; CS = contrast sensitivity; DM = diabetes mellitus; DME = diabetic macular edema; DR = diabetic retinopathy; DTSQ = Diabetes Treatment Satisfaction Questionnaire; ERM = epiretinal membrane; ETDRS = Early Treatment Diabetic Retinopathy Research Group; hx = history; LTF = lost to followup; MH = macular hole; mo = month; NPDR = non proliferative diabetic retinopathy; NR = not reported; OCT = optical coherence tomography; PDR = proliferative diabetic retinopathy; pt = patient; QOL = quality of life; RD = rhegmatogenous retinal detachment; RBX = Ruboxistaurin; T1D = type 1 diabetes mellitus; T2D = type 2 diabetes mellitus; tx = treatment; VA = visual acuity; VF = visual function; VFQ–25 = National Eye Institute Visual Function Questionnaire-25; yr = year(s)

Appendix F. Extended study characteristics and outcomes for studies reporting the impact of interventions for diabetic retinopathy on HRQL (continued)

Study	Study Characteristics	Study Population	HRQL Instrument(s)	Results
Okamoto, 2010[40] **Country:** Japan **Date of study:** June 2005 to April 2007 **Study setting:** outpatient clinic	**Study design:** prospective cohort **Inclusion criteria:** indications for vitrectomy in: G1—PDR: recurrent or persistent nonclearing vitreous hemorrhage, traction, or combined traction-rhegmatogenous RD and adherent posterior hyaloid causing excessive macular traction; G2—DME: clinically significant according to ETDRS guidelines and when ≥ 3 mo had passed after ≥1 session of laser tx and when logMAR BCVA in the affected eye was 0.2 or worse **Exclusion criteria:** 1) pt with hx of vitreoretinal surgery and ocular disorders except for mild refractive errors and mild cataract; 2) pt who had undergone bilateral vitrectomy within 3 mo **Intervention (n):** G1& G2—received pars plana vitrectomy G3—normal controls (100)	**Total population (n):** 399 **Total eyes in study (n):** 399 **Withdrew (n):** 0 **Analyzed n (%):** 399 (100) **Age, mean±SD(range):** G1—57.7±12.9; G2—62.7±9.0 **Males n (%):** G1—53 (13.3); G2—23 (5.8) **Type of DM n (%):** NR **Visual acuity:** G1—BCVA: 1.37±0.75; CS: 5.4±7.2 G2—BCVA: 0.76±0.49; CS: 9.2±6.5 **DR n (%):** 99 (24.8) **Type of DR n (%):** PDR—99 (100) **Other included retinal diseases n (%):** DME—38 (9.5); BRVO—20 (5.0); CRVO—12 (3.0); MH—42 (10.5); ERM—33 (8.3); RD—55 (13.8)	**Instrument/technique:** VFQ–25 **Method of administration:** VFQ–25—self-completed with instructions and assistance from research staff **Respondent:** Pt **Time points of administration:** before and 3 mo after tx **Baseline score mean±SD(range):** G1—52.8±19.0; G2—53.0±20.5	*VFQ–25 (mean±SD)* G1—63.6±17.5; G2—59.0±21.0 *VA (mean±SD)* G1—BCVA: 0.53±0.62; p<0.0001; CS: 14.0±7.9; p<0.0001 G2—BCVA: 0.55±0.51; p<0.001; CS: 12.7±7.1; p<0.0001

ARMD = age-related macular degeneration; BCVA = best corrected visual acuity; BRVO = branch retinal vein occlusion; CRVO = central retinal vein occlusion; CS = contrast sensitivity; DM = diabetes mellitus; DME = diabetic macular edema; DR = diabetic retinopathy; DTSQ = Diabetes Treatment Satisfaction Questionnaire = DTSQ; ERM = epiretinal membrane; ETDRS = Early Treatment Diabetic Retinopathy Research Group; hx = history; LTF = lost to followup; MH = macular hole; mo = month; NPDR = non proliferative diabetic retinopathy; NR = not reported; OCT = optical coherence tomography; PDR = proliferative diabetic retinopathy; pt = patient; QOL = quality of life; RD = rhegmatogenous retinal detachment; RBX = Ruboxistaurin; T1D = type 1 diabetes mellitus; T2D = type 2 diabetes mellitus; tx = treatment; VA = visual acuity; VF = visual function; VFQ–25 = National Eye Institute Visual Function Questionnaire-25; yr = year(s)

Appendix F. Extended study characteristics and outcomes for studies reporting the impact of interventions for diabetic retinopathy on HRQL (continued)

Vitrectomy and panretinal photocoagulation

Study	Study Characteristics	Study Population	HRQL Instrument(s)	Results
Emi, 2009[43] Country: Japan Date of study: NR Study setting: outpatient clinic	Study design: cohort Inclusion criteria: NR Exclusion criteria: NR Intervention (n): G1—no DR: no treatment (131) G2—simple DR: photocoagulation, laser surgery (60) G3—PDR: par plana vitrectomy (136)	Total population (n): 327 Total eyes in study (n): NR Withdrew (n): 0 (0) Analyzed n (%): 327 (100%) Age, mean±SD(range): G1—62.7 (10.0) G2—60.6 (10.1) G3—59.6 (9.6) Males n (%): G1—89 (67.9) G2—39 (65.0) G3—80 (58.8) Type of DM n (%): NR Visual acuity: logMAR (mean): G1—right eye: 1.09; left eye: 1.1; G2—right eye: 0.64; left eye: 0.61; G3—right eye: 0.21; left eye: 0.19 DR n (%): 196 (60) Type of DR n (%): simple DR: 60 (18.3); PDR: 136 (41.6) Other included retinal diseases n (%): NR	Instrument/technique: VFQ-25 Time points of administration: VFQ-25—baseline; 1 yr after tx Baseline score mean±SD(range): VFQ-25 scores, per item: G1—Item 1: 43; Item 2: 73; Item 3: 95; Item 4: 85; Item 5: 93; Item 6: 97; Item 7: 92; Item 8: 93; Item 9: 98; Item 10: 90; Item 11: 98; Item 12: 91 G2—Item 1: 39; Item 2: 58; Item 3: 90; Item 4: 68; Item 5: 84; Item 6: 90; Item 7: 76; Item 8: 78; Item 9: 87; Item 10: 78; Item 11: 92; Item 12: 89 G3—Item 1: 40; Item 2: 43; Item 3: 92; Item 4: 51; Item 5: 64; Item 6: 78; Item 7: 58; Item 8: 71; Item 9: 75; Item 10: 46; Item 11: 89; Item 12: 73	VFQ-25 1 yr scores per item (mean): G1—Item 1: 49; Item 2: 75; Item 3: 94; Item 4: 86; Item 5: 93; Item 6: 98; Item 7: 92; Item 8: 93; Item 9: 99; Item 10: 90; Item 11: 100; Item 12: 90 G2—Item 1: 41; Item 2: 60; Item 3: 89; Item 4: 66; Item 5: 80; Item 6: 88; Item 7: 70; Item 8: 70; Item 9: 83; Item 10: 76; Item 11: 92; Item 12: 84 G3—Item 1: 42; Item 2: 61; Item 3: 88; Item 4: 61; Item 5: 77; Item 6: 82; Item 7: 70; Item 8: 73; Item 9: 81; Item 10: 60; Item 11: 92; Item 12: 78

ARMD = age-related macular degeneration; BCVA = best corrected visual acuity; BRVO = branch retinal vein occlusion; CRVO = central retinal vein occlusion; CS = contrast sensitivity; DM = diabetes mellitus; DME = diabetic macular edema; DR = diabetic retinopathy; DTSQ = Diabetes Treatment Satisfaction Questionnaire; ERM = epiretinal membrane; ETDRS = Early Treatment Diabetic Retinopathy Research Group; hx = history; LTF = lost to followup; MH = macular hole; mo = month; NPDR = non proliferative diabetic retinopathy; NR = not reported; OCT = optical coherence tomography; PDR = proliferative diabetic retinopathy; pt = patient; QOL = quality of life; RD = rhegmatogenous retinal detachment; RBX = Ruboxistaurin; T1D = type 1 diabetes mellitus; T2D = type 2 diabetes mellitus; tx = treatment; VA = visual acuity; VF = visual function; VFQ-25 = National Eye Institute Visual Function Questionnaire-25; yr = year(s)

Appendix F. Extended study characteristics and outcomes for studies reporting the impact of interventions for diabetic retinopathy on HRQL (continued)

Study	Study Characteristics	Study Population	HRQL Instrument(s)	Results
Phacoemulsification cataract surgery				
Mozaffarieh, 2005a[49] Country: Austria Date of study: May 2001 to May 2003 Study setting: outpatient clinic	Study design: prospective cohort Inclusion criteria: 1) undergoing standardized first-eye phacoemulsification cataract surgery Exclusion criteria: 1) pt dx with glaucoma, uveitis, hx of ocular trauma or any other co-existing, visually limiting condition other than those associated with DR; 2) pt with a progression of DR in the non-operated fellow eye Intervention (n): G1—pt with no apparent retinopathy (17) G2—pt with mild NPDR (19) G3—pt with severe NPDR (16) G4—pt with PDR (15) All groups—received phacoemulsification cataract surgery	Total population (n): 74 Total eyes in study (n): 74 Withdrew (n): died (1), did not complete/return questionnaire (6) Analyzed n (%): 67 (90.5) Age, mean±SD(range): 57.8 (42–68) (all); G1–57.9 (48–67); G2–55.5 (42–66); G3–59.1 (49–67); G4–59.1 (44–71) Males n (%): NR Type of DM n (%): T2D–65 (97) Visual acuity: mean (range) G1—Snellen: 0.29 (0.05–0.50); logMAR VA: 0.62 (0.30–1.30); G2—Snellen: 0.29 (0.05–0.50); logMAR VA: 0.60 (0.30–1.30); G3—Snellen: 0.28 (0.05–0.50); logMAR VA: 0.67 (0.30–1.30); G4—Snellen: 0.24 (0.05–0.40); logMAR VA: 0.71 (0.40–1.30) DR n (%): 50 (74.6) Type of DR n (%): mild NPDR 19 (28.3); severe NPDR 16 (23.9); PDR 15 (22.4) Other included retinal diseases n (%): 3 patients with severe NPDR had DME	Instrument/technique: VF-14; patient satisfaction questionnaire Time points of administration: VF-14—before and 3 mo after tx; Snellen chart—before and 3 mo after tx; Patient satisfaction questionnaire—3 mo after tx Baseline score mean±SD(range): VF-14: G1–52.21 (32.14–78.57); G2–55.92 (30.36–85.71); G3–46.65 (30.36–64.29); G4–40.12 (25.00–67.86)	VF-14 (mean [range]) G1–94.54 (85.71–100) G2–91.92 (62.50–100) G3–55.92 (41.07–69.64) G4–45.12 (0–78.57) Patient satisfaction—65.7% of pt completely satisfied G1–82.4% G2–79.0% G3–56.3% G4–40%; surgery met expectations— G1–70.6% G2–73.6% G3–31.2% G4–26.6% Visual Acuity (mean [range]) G1—Snellen: 0.85 (0.60–1.00); logMAR VA: 0.07 (0–0.22); G2—Snellen: 0.80 (0.50–1.00); logMAR VA: 0.10 (0–0.30); G3—Snellen: 0.49 (0.10–0.70); logMAR VA: 0.40 (0.15–1.00); G4—Snellen: 0.37 (0.01–0.60); logMAR VA: 0.56 (0.22–2.00)

ARMD = age-related macular degeneration; BCVA = best corrected visual acuity; BRVO = branch retinal vein occlusion; CRVO = central retinal vein occlusion; CS = contrast sensitivity; DM = diabetes mellitus; DME = diabetic macular edema; DR = diabetic retinopathy; DTSQ = Diabetes Treatment Satisfaction Questionnaire; ERM = epiretinal membrane; ETDRS = Early Treatment Diabetic Retinopathy Research Group; hx = history; LTF = lost to followup; MH = macular hole; mo = month; NPDR = non proliferative diabetic retinopathy; NR = not reported; OCT = optical coherence tomography; PDR = proliferative diabetic retinopathy; pt = patient; QOL = quality of life; RD = rhegmatogenous retinal detachment; RBX = Ruboxistaurin; T1D = type 1 diabetes mellitus; T2D = type 2 diabetes mellitus; tx = treatment; VA = visual acuity; VF = visual function; VFQ-25 = National Eye Institute Visual Function Questionnaire-25; yr = year(s)

Appendix F. Extended study characteristics and outcomes for studies reporting the impact of interventions for diabetic retinopathy on HRQL (continued)

Study	Study Characteristics	Study Population	HRQL Instrument(s)	Results
Mozaffarieh, 2009[47] **Country:** Austria **Date of study:** NR **Study setting:** outpatient clinic	**Study design:** prospective cohort **Inclusion criteria:** 1) presence of bilateral cataract **Exclusion criteria:** 2) pt in whom lenticular opacity did not allow accurate diagnosis of preoperative level of DR; 2) pt with glaucoma, uveitis, hx of ocular trauma or any other coexisting, visually limiting condition; 3) level of DR in the fellow eye was different from first eye at the 6 mo followup **Intervention (n):** G1—pt treated with a single surgery (41) G2—pt treated with a second surgery (48) *Both groups:* phacoemulsification cataract surgery	**Total population (n):** 102 **Total eyes in study (n):** **Withdrew (n):** died (2), lost to followup (7), excluded at 6 mo (4) **Analyzed n (%):** 89 (87.3) **Age, mean±SD(range):** 63.5 (49–78) (total) G1—56.9 G2—58.9 **Males n (%):** 49 (55.1) (total) G1—24 (58.6) G2—25 (52) **Type of DM n (%):** NR **Visual acuity:** NR **DR n (%):** 66 (74.2) **Type of DR n (%):** mild DR—23 (25.8); moderate DR—22 (24.7); PDR—21 (23.6) **Other included retinal diseases n (%):** 1 patient with moderate DR had DME	**Instrument/technique:** VF-14 **Time points of administration:** VF-14—before tx, 1, 3, 6, 8, 12 mo after tx **Baseline score mean±SD(range):** G1—No DR: 69.3±12.4; mild NPDR: 39.3±5.2; severe NPDR: 40.9±8.6; PDR: 35.3±4.4 G2—No DR: 46.8±8.7; mild NPDR: 63.4±16.3; severe NPDR: 50.6±11.4	*VF-14(mean±SD)*— *G1* 1 mo—no DR: 97.1±2.6; mild NPDR: 86.7±14.2; severe NPDR: 40.9±8.6; PDR: 36.3±3.9 3 mo—no DR: 97.1±2.6; mild NPDR: 86.7±14.2; severe NPDR: 50.2±6.4; PDR: 38.1±14.9 6 mo—no DR: 96.8±2.0; mild NPDR: 86.5±13.6; severe NPDR: 48.8±6.7; PDR: 37.9±14.0 8 mo—no DR: 79.5±5.5; mild NPDR: 73.2±8.1; severe NPDR: 47.7±10.4; PDR: 41.5±9.8 12 mo—no DR: 79.5±5.5; mild NPDR: 72.2±8.3; severe NPDR: 46.1±10.7; PDR: 39.9±9.0 *G2* 1 mo—no DR: 93.3±4.2; mild NPDR: 96.4±2.3; severe NPDR: 54.6±8.7; PDR: 49.2±10.9 3 mo—no DR: 93.4±4.3; mild NPDR: 96.4±2.3; severe NPDR: 61.2±6.4; PDR: 57.1±11.6 6 mo—no DR: 93.0±4.3; mild NPDR: 94.6±2.5; severe NPDR: 60.9 6.6; PDR: 53.0±10.9 8 mo—no DR: 93.5±3.1; mild NPDR: 95.9±3.5; severe NPDR: 50.9±16.3; PDR: 53.8±17.6 12 mo—no DR: 95.3±1.9; mild NPDR: 95.3±2.2; severe NPDR: 47.8±16.0; PDR: 47.6±15.0

ARMD = age-related macular degeneration; BCVA = best corrected visual acuity; BRVO = branch retinal vein occlusion; CRVO = central retinal vein occlusion; CS = contrast sensitivity; DM = diabetes mellitus; DME = diabetic macular edema; DR = diabetic retinopathy; DRG = Diabetic Retinopathy Research Group; hx = history; LTF = lost to followup; MH = macular hole; mo = month; NPDR = non proliferative diabetic retinopathy; NR = not reported; OCT = optical coherence tomography; PDR = proliferative diabetic retinopathy; pt = patient; QOL = quality of life; RD = rhegmatogenous retinal detachment; RBX = Ruboxistaurin; T1D = type 1 diabetes mellitus; T2D = type 2 diabetes mellitus; tx = treatment; VA = visual acuity; VF = visual function; VFQ-25 = National Eye Institute Visual Function Questionnaire-25; yr = year(s)

Study	Study Characteristics	Study Population	HRQL Instrument(s)	Results
Anti-VEGF				
Mitchell 2011 Multicenter (73 centers in Australia, Canada, Europe and Turkey) **Date of study:** NR **Study name:** RESTORE	**Study design:** RCT **Inclusion criteria:** ≥18 years with either type 1 or type 2 diabetes mellitus; HbA1c ≤ 10%; stable medication for management of DM; visual impairment due to DME in ≥1 eye that was eligible for laser tx; BCVA between 78–39 (20/32–20/160 Snellen); decreased vision not due to other causes than DME **Exclusion criteria:** concomitant conditions preventing vision improvement; active inflammation in other eye; uncontrolled glaucoma; panretinal laser photocoagulation (w/ in 6 mo) or focal/grid laser photocoagulation (w/ in 3 mo); antiangiogenic drugs w/in 3 mo; hx of stroke, hypertension or change in hypertensive tx (w/ in 3 mo) **Intervention (n):** *G1*—**ranibizumab 0.5 mg + sham laser** (116) *G2*—**ranibizumab 0.5 mg + laser** (118) *G3*—**laser + sham injection** (111)	**Total population (n):** 345 **Total eyes in study (n):** 345 Randomized: 345 Withdrew (n): 42 Analyzed [HRQL at 12 mo] (n; %) 303 (88) **Age, mean±SD:** *G1*—62.9±9.29 *G2*—64.0±8.15 *G3*—63.5±8.81 **Males n (%):** *G1*—73 (63) *G2*—70 (59) *G3*—58 (52) **Type of DM n (%):** T1D—41 (12); T2D—302 (88); unknown—2 (<1) **VA (letter score), mean±SD:** *G1*—64.8±10.11 *G2*—63.4±9.99 *G3*—62.4±11.11 **Type of DME n (%):** *Focal*—185 (54) *Diffuse*—143 (41) *Unknown*—17 (5)	**Instrument:** NEI-VFQ-25 **Method of administration:** NR **Respondent:** Pt **Time points of administration:** baseline, 3 mo, 12 mo **Baseline score, mean±SD:** *NEI-VFQ-25* *G1*—NR *G2*—NR *G3*—NR	*VFQ-25, composite score at 12 mo* *G1*—baseline: NR; improvement: 5.0 *G2*—baseline: NR; improvement: 5.4 *G3*—baseline: NR; improvement: 0.6 *VFQ-25, subscales at 12 mo* General vision *G1*—baseline: NR; improvement: 8.9 *G2*—baseline: NR; improvement: 8.0 *G3*—baseline: NR; improvement: 1.1 Distance activities *G1*—baseline: NR; improvement: 5.3 *G2*—baseline: NR; improvement: 5.6 *G3*—baseline: NR; improvement: 0.4 Near activities *G1*—baseline: NR; improvement: 9.0 *G2*—baseline: NR; improvement: 9.1 *G3*—baseline: NR; improvement: 1.1 Remaining vision related subscales—NR

BCVA = best corrected visual acuity; BRVO = branch retinal vein occlusion; CRVO = central retinal vein occlusion; CS = contrast sensitivity; CSMO = Clinically Significant Macular oedema; DM = diabetes mellitus; DME = diabetic macular edema; DR = diabetic retinopathy; ETDRS = Early Treatment Diabetic Retinopathy Research Group; hx = history; LTF = lost to followup;; mo = month; NPDR = non proliferative diabetic retinopathy; NR = not reported; OCT = optical coherence tomography; PDR = proliferative diabetic retinopathy; pt = patient; QOL = quality of life; T1D = type 1 diabetes mellitus; T2D = type 2 diabetes mellitus; tx = treatment; VA = visual acuity; VF = visual function; VFQ-25 = National Eye Institute Visual Function Questionnaire-25; yr = year(s)

Study	Study Characteristics	Study Population	HRQL Instrument(s)	Results
Sultan 2011 Multicenter (60 centers in Australia, Europe, India, North America, South America) Date of study: Sep 2005 – Nov 2009 Study name: Macugen 1013	Study design: RCT Inclusion criteria: ≥18 yr; DME involving center of the macula not assoc with ischemia; foveal thickness ≥250µm; BCVA 65-35 (20/50–20/200 Snellen); intraocular pressure ≤21mmHg; clear ocular media; adequate papillary dilation, hematologic, liver & renal function Exclusion criteria: any abnormality likely to confound assessment of VA; atrophy/scarring/fibrosis of center of macula; subfoveal hard exudates or retinal pigment epithelial atrophy; YAG laser, peripheral retinal cryoablation, laser retinopexy, focal or grid photocoagulation within prior 16 wk; panretinal photocoagulation within prior 6 mo or needed within in 9 mo; intraocular surgery within in 6 prior mo; hx of vitrectomy; previous filtering surgery or placement of drainage device; significant media opacities; pathologic high myopia; prior radiation in region of study eye; uncontrolled DM Intervention (n): G1—pegaptanib 0.3 mg (133) G2—sham injection (127)	Total population (n): 288 Total eyes in study (n): 288 Withdrew (n): 28 (at wk 54); 95 (at wk 102) Analyzed [HRQL, 54 wk] n (%):260 (90) Age, mean±SD: G1—62.3±9.3 G2—62.5±10.2 Males n (%): G1—81 (61) G2—68 (54) Type of DM n (%):T1D—18 (7); T2D—242 (93) VA (letter score), mean±SD: G1—57.0±8.9 G2—57.5±8.1 Type of DME n (%): 100 (100%)	Instrument/technique: NEI-VFQ-25 Method of administration: in person in India; via telephone for all other centers Respondent: Pt Time points of administration: baseline, 18, 54 & 102 wk Baseline score mean±SD(range): NEI-VFQ-25 G1—65.9 G2—67.9	*VFQ-25, composite score at 54 wk:* G1—70.4; improvement 4.5 G2—69.2; improvement 1.3 *Between group differences*— 2.92; range -0.32 to 6.16 (p = 0.077) *VFQ-25 subscales at 54 wk:* Near vision activities—between group differences: 5.70; 0.48-10.91 (p = 0.033) Distance vision functioning—between group differences: 8.50; 2.74-14.25 (p = 0.044) Social functioning—between group differences: 7.99; 2.90-13.09 (p = 0.002) Between group differences were not statistically significant for the 8 remaining vision related subscales *VFQ-25, composite score at 102 wk (n = 207):* G1—69.8; improvement 4.6 G2—66.2; improvement 0.1 *Between group differences*— 4.47; range -0.26 to 8.68 (p = 0.038)

BCVA = best corrected visual acuity; BRVO = branch retinal vein occlusion; CRVO = central retinal vein occlusion; CS = contrast sensitivity; CSMO = Clinically Significant Macular oedema; DM = diabetes mellitus; DME = diabetic macular edema; DR = diabetic retinopathy; ETDRS = Early Treatment Diabetic Retinopathy Research Group; hx = history; LTF = lost to followup;: mo = month; NPDR = non proliferative diabetic retinopathy; NR = not reported; OCT = optical coherence tomography; PDR = proliferative diabetic retinopathy; pt = patient; QOL = quality of life; T1D = type 1 diabetes mellitus; T2D = type 2 diabetes mellitus; tx = treatment; VA = visual acuity; VF = visual function; VFQ-25 = National Eye Institute Visual Function Questionnaire-25; yr = year(s)